Advance praise for
The X-ray Information Book

Dr. Laws's book helps the consumer to put into clear perspective the benefits and risks associated with medical X-rays. It offers practical suggestions on how to avoid unnecessary exposure, and should help to foster a constructive dialogue between physician and patient about whether or not X-rays are needed. Perhaps most important, this book is notably free of the near-hysteria about radiation dangers that characterizes so much recent writing on the subject.

—John C. Villforth, Director
National Center for Devices and
Radiological Health
FOOD AND DRUG ADMINISTRATION

THE X-RAY
INFORMATION
BOOK

THE X-RAY INFORMATION BOOK

A Consumers' Guide to Avoiding

Unnecessary Medical and

Dental X-rays

Priscilla W. Laws, Ph.D., and

The Public Citizen Health

Research Group

Foreword by Sidney M. Wolfe, M.D.

Farrar · Straus · Giroux
New York

Revised edition of *Medical and Dental X-rays: A Consumers' Guide to
Avoiding Unnecessary Radiation Exposure.* Portions of *The X-ray Information Book* previously appeared in *X-rays: More Harm Than Good?*
published by Rodale Press; copyright © 1977 by Priscilla W. Laws

Library of Congress Cataloging in Publication Data
Laws, Priscilla W.
The X-ray information book.
Rev. ed. of: Medical and dental X-rays. 1974.
Includes bibliographical references.
1. Diagnosis, Radioscopic—Complications and sequelae.
2. X-rays—Physiological effect.   3. X-rays—Safety
measures.   4. Consumer protection.   I. Public Citizen, Inc.
Health Research Group.   II. Title.
RC78.L36   1983   616.07'572   82-20923

ACKNOWLEDGMENTS

This book would not have been possible without the inspiration provided by Dr. Sidney Wolfe, M.D., and his fine staff at Public Citizen Health Research Group in Washington, D.C. It was the Health Research Group's profound belief in the power of informed consumers to effect change that motivated the original consumers' guide on which this book is based.

I am grateful to Mark Barnett, MPH; Joseph Arcarese, MS; James Benson, MS; and Jim Morrison of the Bureau of Radiological Health; Otha Linton, of the Washington Office of the American College of Radiology; and Robert Gorson, MS, of Jefferson Medical College for providing me with basic information about diagnostic X-rays and for reviewing parts of this book or the original consumers' guide. Radiologists John Harris, Jr., Theodore Bledsoe, and Albert Herwit, and my present family dentist, G. Ronald Krajack, provided invaluable comments about the practical side of conducting diagnostic X-ray examinations. Although these professionals did not always agree with my conclusions about diagnostic X-ray use, I appreciated their input.

Wendy Cheyfitz, Marcia Conner, and Frances Wat-

Acknowledgments

son, among others, provided editorial help and laymen's reactions to parts of the manuscript.

Finally, I would like to thank the several hundred "patients" throughout the United States who wrote me about their actual diagnostic X-ray experiences.

Priscilla W. Laws
Carlisle, Pa.

NOTE TO THE READER

This book is primarily about X-rays used for diagnostic purposes. Diagnostic X-rays help physicians and dentists locate conditions in the human body which can cause illness.

X-rays are also used for therapeutic purposes to kill cancerous cells, to destroy ringworm and other fungi, and to treat acne. Nuclear scans are sometimes used in which radioactive substances that give off X-rays and other particles are introduced into the body for diagnostic purposes. Although these uses of radiation in health care also involve expense and exposure, they are not nearly so widespread as the use of diagnostic X-rays. Therapeutic X-rays and nuclear scans will, I hope, be the subject of other writings for consumers.

CONTENTS

Contents

FOREWORD

The dangerous gap between what the doctor knows and what the patient knows is getting smaller. During the 1970s, consumers started becoming aware of some of the risks of medical waste both to their health and to their pocketbooks. Needless surgery, overprescribing of drugs, unnecessary hospitalizations, and overbuilding of hospital facilities not only waste billions of dollars but also lead each year to worse health care and tens of thousands of deaths and injuries that could have been avoided. Although at the beginning of the 1970s each of these excesses seemed out of control, there has recently been a major turnaround, mainly because of increased awareness and individual and collective action by the victims of these dangerous medical practices and by the families of those who have died as a result of such practices. For example:

• Since the mid-1970s there has been a steady decrease in the overall number of prescriptions filled in the United States, especially for such overprescribed categories as sleeping pills, tranquilizers, menopausal estrogens, and cholesterol-lowering drugs.

• Many formerly overprescribed surgical procedures, such as tonsillectomies and hysterectomies, are being performed less frequently.

• Some patients who formerly would have been hospitalized automatically are now being treated as outpatients, with better results and at lower cost.

The more we learn about the dangers of radiation to our bodies—especially cancer and genetic damage— the clearer it becomes that consumer health action on yet another front may be necessary.

Updates of 1979 Food and Drug Administration information[1] show that in 1982:

• One hundred fifty-four million Americans— seven out of every ten people—received at least one medical or dental X-ray exam, for a total of 312 million X-ray examinations that year.

• Assuming a conservatively low average cost of $20 per dental X-ray exam and $50 per medical X-ray exam, over $12.5 billion dollars was spent in 1982 on diagnostic X-rays in the United States.

If all this radiation exposure was necessary and without risk, there would be no need to question such massive expenditures. As Dr. Priscilla Laws has documented in this book, however, this is not the case.

No one would dispute the fact that the use of certain drugs, operations, or other procedures to treat or diagnose particular diseases is justifiable, even though fraught with a certain amount of risk. Similarly, diagnostic X-rays, properly and appropriately done, are an important part of the practice of medicine and dentistry.

But what about X-rays that should not have been done at all or ones that were done with poorly functioning equipment, poor techniques, and/or inadequate patient protection? In each case, the patient is the victim of unnecessary radiation and its attendant hazards.

Several years ago, Dr. Laws, a Professor of Physics at Dickinson College, wrote to Public Citizens' Health Research Group concerning the problem of medical and dental X-ray exposure.

Recently I asked my dentist what dose I would receive from the routine X-ray examinations he conducts every 6 months. He became very angry and said that I had no right to question his professional competence. In fact, if I planned to use the dosage information to decide whether I ought to have X-rays, I could find another dentist. He would not release any data to me.

Dr. Laws expressed further concern about the lack of any federal or state regulations for control of cumulative medical and dental X-ray doses received by an individual and about the lack of consumer awareness of the risks involved. She offered to work on these problems with us during her sabbatical leave the following year. We gladly accepted, and this book is one product of that effort.

The arrogance of many health professionals toward legitimate consumer concerns about radiation exposure (a major factor in the genesis of this book) can be seen in raw form in a letter from a radiologist who reviewed the manuscript for this book: "As a matter of general philosophy, I resent the intrusion of consumerism into the practice of medicine, especially when the physician's judgment is called into question." Because of this condescending "don't question my judgment" attitude of many doctors toward consumers, which represents the most unhealthy aspect of the doctor-patient relationship, it is particularly essential for patients to initiate questions about what doctors are planning to do.

Poor judgment on the part of physicians and dentists is only one of many factors contributing to unnecessary X-ray exposures. Other major factors include X-ray examinations conducted primarily for the legal protection of practitioners, the use of poor or outdated equipment, and the use of sloppy techniques by those responsible for taking X-rays.

A look at the results of a few recent studies reveals the enormity of this problem:

Foreword

Former National Cancer Institute Director Dr. Arthur Upton has recently estimated that diagnostic X-rays cause approximately 3,670 cancer deaths per year in the United States and an incalculable amount of genetic damage.[2]

An estimated 30 percent of diagnostic X-ray procedures are unnecessary[3]—if you include exams that should never have been ordered in the first place and unnecessary X-rays due to retakes—and an additional estimated one-third of the radiation dose could be avoided, even for necessary X-rays, if radiation exposure were limited to the size of the film.[4] Therefore, *at least half the diagnostic X-radiation dose being absorbed by American health consumers is an expensive, unnecessary danger* resulting in a wasteful expenditure of at least $3.75 billion dollars a year (30 percent unnecessary procedures times $12.5 billion total X-ray bill) and causing at least 1,800 preventable cases of X-radiation-induced cancer a year (50 percent unnecessary radiation exposure times 3,670 radiation-induced cancer deaths a year).

Some of the causes of this damage are stated below.

• One out of five X-ray units checked by state radiation inspectors in 1980 were not in compliance with state law,[5] often causing patients to be exposed to excessive and illegal amounts of radiation emitted from faulty equipment.

• Nonradiologist physicians who own their own X-ray machines use twice as many X-ray examinations as colleagues who refer their patients to radiologists.[4]

• A national survey of dental X-ray exposure showed that some X-rays gave eighty times more radiation to the patient than others.[6] Similar ranges of exposure have been seen for medical X-rays.

• As many as 10 percent of medical X-ray films have to be repeated because of poor technique, thus amounting to over fifty million wasted X-ray films (and radiation doses) per year.[7]

• X-rays ordered for legal, not medical, purposes (to protect the doctor rather than the patient) can be greatly reduced—as indicated by a 40 percent reduction in skull X-rays for head-trauma patients after an "educational" program for doctors was started without causing adverse outcomes in those who did not get an X-ray.[8]

Considering how serious the problem of unnecessary X-radiation is, you need to protect yourself by asking more questions any time someone suggests you need an X-ray and by demanding reasonable answers to your questions.

This book explains what X-rays are, how they can harm you, and what the major sources of unnecessary exposure are. It concludes with a description of some practical steps consumers can take to reduce unnecessary X-ray exposure and still obtain positive benefits from diagnostic X-ray examinations.

Sidney M. Wolfe, M.D.
Director
Public Citizen Health Research Group

THE X-RAY
INFORMATION
BOOK

CHAPTER

I

Introduction

Medical and dental X-rays provide a powerful tool in the diagnosis and treatment of injury, disease, and other conditions that influence human health. Although one purpose of this book is to dispel the myth that diagnostic X-ray examinations are beneficial under all circumstances, the major purpose is to outline steps that can be taken by informed consumers to minimize the risks associated with unneeded exposure to diagnostic X-rays without reducing the substantial benefits of diagnostic X-ray examinations.

Public awareness of the dangers of exposure to radiation has come a long way since Wilhelm C. Roentgen discovered the X-ray in 1895. Slowly but steadily the dangers of X-rays and similar kinds of radiation have been recognized. The myth that small amounts of radium salts taken internally had positive medicinal properties was quickly dispelled. Similarly, shoe store fluoroscopes, used to view the foot bones of millions of children while unknowingly exposing them to X-rays in the 1940s and 1950s, have fortunately disappeared from the scene. The use of the first atomic bombs in 1945 demonstrated the direct and devastating effects of high levels of radiation. Studies on fallout from the large-scale testing of nuclear weapons in the late 1950s and early 1960s raised concern about the effects on human populations of adding relatively low levels of radiation to the global environment. Studies of children whose mothers were exposed to medical X-rays during pregnancy, of adults who received diagnostic X-ray examinations, and of laboratory experiments on animals have all contributed to our understanding of how low levels of radiation adversely affect humans. It is currently believed that exposure to low-level radiation may increase an individual's chance of having damaged genes, a shorter life, cancer, or leukemia.

Although some radiation has always been part of the natural environment, in recent years a number of human activities have served to approximately double the amount of radiation to which the average person is exposed. In addition to fallout from testing nuclear weapons, activities such as watching television, wearing radium-dial watches, and flying at high altitudes in jet airplanes have increased the amount of radiation humans absorb. At present there is a major controversy about the risks associated with the low-level radiation released to the environment from nuclear power plants. In spite of the degree of public awareness about nuclear power plants and fallout as threats to public health, many people do not realize that *diagnostic X-rays currently constitute the largest source of man-made radiation exposure to the U.S. population.*

Because it is recognized that exposure to any amount of radiation is potentially harmful, government agencies and advisory groups have set guidelines limiting doses individuals working near radiation can receive annually. Guidelines have also been set limiting the amount of man-made radiation to which the general public can be exposed. However, because no regulatory agency or advisory group places any restrictions on the exposure received by patients from X-ray examinations, *it is possible for a complete series of diagnostic abdominal X-ray examinations received by a patient in any year to exceed the annual occupational limit for radiation dose.*

Although most physicians believe that the overall benefits of the diagnostic X-ray examinations probably outweigh the risks, an increasing number of professionals feel that diagnostic X-rays are often misused and overused by medical and dental practitioners. For example, a report published by the Environmental

Protection Agency states that ". . . it appears reasonable that as much as a 50% reduction in dose might be possible due to [improvement in] technical and educational methods."[1] John Villforth, director of the Bureau of Radiological Health of the Food and Drug Administration, has estimated that as many as 30 percent of all diagnostic X-ray procedures may be unnecessary.[2] It is estimated that for all X-rays one-third of the radiation dose could be avoided if exposure to the X-ray beam is consistently limited to the size of the film.[3] Regardless of whether or not these estimates are accurate, many qualified professionals feel that a significant portion of the present annual population exposure to diagnostic X-rays is unnecessary.

The American College of Radiology has taken the position that in diagnostic radiology the goal is to obtain the desired information using the smallest radiation exposure that is practical.[4] Any additional exposure is unnecessary and is certainly more harmful than beneficial. This commendable goal has not yet been attained because many physicians and other health personnel who order or perform X-ray examinations have not been sufficiently concerned about the hazards of radiation. Thus it is especially important for consumers to make sure, whenever possible, that the risks associated with each diagnostic X-ray examination are minimized and that the examination is not conducted unless its potential benefits outweigh the associated risks.

CHAPTER

II

Misuses of
Diagnostic X-rays

There are three major causes of unnecessary exposure to medical and dental X-rays. One cause can be traced to poor judgment on the part of practitioners, employers, and/or patients about the real medical benefits of particular X-ray examinations. Another significant cause of wasted X-rays can be traced to medical and dental professionals' use of X-rays for the purpose of defending themselves in possible malpractice suits. The third major cause of unnecessary X-rays is use of poor equipment and/or sloppy techniques by those responsible for conducting X-ray examinations. Details on how individual consumers can reduce their exposure to unnecessary X-rays are contained in Chapter VI of this guide.

When a physician or a dentist examines a patient with certain symptoms, it is his or her responsibility to determine what additional information is needed to establish the correct diagnosis. Ideally the decision to use X-rays is based on some clinical indication that the patient may have a condition that can be accurately diagnosed only with an appropriate X-ray examination. A clinical indication is based on tangible evidence the examining physician or dentist can see, feel, or hear, or on information about a patient's background, age, or medical history. Unfortunately many X-rays have been wasted on people because decisions to use them have been motivated by factors not related to the health of the patient.

According to Dr. Herbert L. Abrams, chairman of the Harvard Medical School Department of Radiology, ignorance of the limitations of diagnostic X-ray examinations and a desire for action and certainty lead practitioners to an undue dependence on X-ray examinations.[1] This overuse of X-rays has probably increased because many X-ray examinations are covered under medical insurance plans, so direct expense to the patient is not a problem. (Everyone who pays premiums on medical insurance bears the costs of these examinations, however.)

Physicians often order X-rays so that they have an X-ray available for legal evidence if a patient files a malpractice suit. The practice of ordering treatments and diagnostic tests for the primary purpose of malpractice protection is known as defensive medicine. This practice seems to be widespread, and 50 percent to 70 percent of physicians who are polled admit to engaging in some form of defensive medicine.[2,3]

A number of courts have ruled, however, that a physician or a dentist may be held negligent for failing to take diagnostic X-rays *only if it is shown that common practice requires the physician to do so in view of the patient's symptoms.*[4,5] It is likely that in many cases where there are no accepted clinical indications that an X-ray diagnosis will be useful, X-rays taken for defensive purposes will provide little protection for either the physician or the patient.

X-ray examinations are often conducted for the legal protection of employers. The most common of these examinations consists of the routine preemployment lower back (lumbar spine) X-ray series for workers doing heavy lifting. Some employers assume that an X-ray examination of the lower back can predict the chances the employee may develop a job-related back disability if structural defects of the spine are detected. Some investigators have found evidence that this is not true.[6]

Although at a conference on preemployment physical examinations[7] it was concluded that routine X-rays of the lower back might have value in assessing the degree of already existing disabilities, clear evidence

9

supporting this contention was not available. Unfortunately, lower-back or lumbar-spine X-rays require higher exposures than almost any other commonly used diagnostic examination. (See Chapter V for details.)

Another common preemployment examination is the chest X-ray required by certain states for job categories such as teaching and food handling. One problem is that photofluorographic X-rays are often used in preemployment screening tests rather than conventional chest X-rays, a procedure that exposes a person to more radiation than an ordinary chest X-ray examination. (See Chapter V for details.)

For many years social agencies offered free mass screening chest X-rays to the public. Countless persons, without consulting their physician, subjected themselves to X-rays in mobile units. Chest X-rays taken in mobile units usually involve significantly more exposure than conventional X-ray machines[8] and risk becomes a more important factor. Although at one time mobile units may have been a necessary part of a viable public health program, tuberculosis has been virtually eradicated from most areas in the United States. Thus, in 1972 the Bureau of Radiological Health, the American College of Radiology, and the American College of Chest Physicians recommended in a joint statement that mass chest X-ray surveys of the general population for tuberculosis and other cardiopulmonary (heart and lung) diseases be discontinued. To screen for tuberculosis, easy-to-perform skin tests can be used instead of chest X-rays. In spite of this recent procedure, a few local Tuberculosis Associations may still encourage screening by urging people to have chest X-ray examinations without consulting with their physicians. Although physicians often make errors in judgment about X-rays, patients probably make even more and should not be referring themselves for X-rays, especially in mobile units. J. L. McClenahan states that "X-rays are commonly used to treat anxiety in patients or in doctors."[9]

Some physicians admit that they will allow an anxious patient to be X-rayed in order to reduce his or her anxiety, without determining whether the screening is needed. Putting the patient's mind at ease and/or fattening their own pocketbooks must seem more important to these doctors than carefully examining the patient in order to decide whether or not an X-ray examination is really needed. Sometimes it might be more appropriate for the doctor to be honest by informing the anxious patient that the doctor can find no indications of a serious problem and that an X-ray will add no useful information to a diagnosis. Ordering X-ray examinations solely for their psychological value in relieving anxiety is similar to the use of placebos as medication. However, unlike some placebos which are harmless, an X-ray examination used as a placebo involves a risk for the patient. Serious questions have been raised about the ethics of using placebos.[10]

Another example of the misuse of X-ray examinations is the executive physical examination. Routinely prescribed by the management of some companies for top executives, the executive physical examination may subject these people, among other dangers, to X-ray examinations of the spine, kidney, and upper and lower gastrointestinal tracts (the GI series). The GI series and lower spinal examinations are among the highest-risk examinations. Although passing an executive physical seems to give many companies and their executives a sense of well-being, there is little evidence that the use of high-risk routine X-ray examinations justifies the benefits.

Dental examinations involve X-ray exposure of a very limited area of the body containing few critical organs. They do not pose as much of a threat to individual health as a number of medical X-ray examinations. Despite this fact, the practice of conducting routine examinations without any clinical indication that they will yield new information is also widespread in dentistry, and can result in significant costs and radiation exposure over a period.

The American Dental Association and other organizations[11,12,13,14] have stated that dental X-ray examinations should not be performed routinely, and that a decision to X-ray should be made only *after* a visual examination of the mouth and a history of the patient are obtained.

Most members of the dental profession feel that it is legitimate to have on file a set of full-mouth X-ray exposures or a panoramic study. Then, unless there is clear evidence of cavities between the teeth or of gum problems, only occasional individual films are needed to check trouble spots. Yet some dentists take full-mouth X-rays much more often than is necessary. Many persons who rarely have cavities or gum problems are subjected to routine bitewing examinations at frequent intervals. The small health risks involved with dental X-rays are probably less significant than the extra expense to which patients are subjected.

Because breast cancer is a leading cause of death in women between the ages of 39 and 44, the American Cancer Society has recommended periodic breast X-ray screening examinations, known as mammograms, for certain women over the age of 35. (See Chapter VI for details.) [15] Unfortunately, the female breast is more prone to radiation-induced cancer than any other organ. One study of the risk-benefit trade-off for mammography published in 1982 concluded that the 1980 American Cancer Society policy calling for annual mammographic examinations beginning in the mid-to-late forties is not justified in view of the accuracy with which diagnoses can be made. [16] The authors recommend biennial mammograms instead.

Although physicians are more aware of the extra danger X-rays pose to unborn children than they were in the past, some practitioners still order routine pelvimetric examinations in order to determine the size of a woman's pelvis. Occasionally physicians have admitted that they are embarrassed to ask a young single woman who requires an X-ray examination that exposes the abdominal area if she might be pregnant. If a pregnancy is suspected it is wise to defer such an examination, if it is possible to do so, until the woman is no longer pregnant and does not expect to become pregnant within three months after the X-ray examination.

Referring specifically to pelvimetry, the practice of X-raying the pelvis of a pregnant woman to determine the size of the birth canal, an expert panel convened by the American College of Obstetricians and Gynecologists and the American College of Radiological Health of the Food and Drug Administration concluded that X-ray pelvimetry should not be considered as "usual and customary" in the practice of obstetrics.[17]

Another source of unproductive exposure to X-rays is the practice of repeating examinations unnecessarily. Although reexaminations are sometimes needed to monitor changes in a condition, physicians and dentists have sometimes been capricious with routine repetitions of the same examination. Hospitals, physicians, and dentists do not always acquire or accept perfectly good X-ray studies conducted at other facilities.

In 1980 a panel of physicians convened by the Department of Health and Human Services stated that the yield of unsuspected disease revealed by routine screening chest X-ray examinations has been of insufficient clinical value to justify the monetary cost, added radiation exposure, and patient inconvenience.[18] Nonetheless, it is still common practice for hospitals to require chest X-rays of all outpatients visiting their X-ray Departments and of all inpatients before admission to the hospital.

At present, the process of deciding whether or not to X-ray usually demands that a physician or a dentist make a subjective professional judgment. The fact that results of an X-ray examination are negative does not necessarily mean the practitioner who requested the study used unsound judgment. Nor do negative results from an X-ray study necessarily mean a person is healthy. However, much more substantial research needs to be conducted to correlate the clinically observable symptoms of a patient with the probability that the results of an examination will yield medically significant information. The information obtained from the diagnosis of a suspected condition is significant if, sooner or later, it changes the plan for the treatment of the patient. Too often X-rays are merely taken to see what's there, rather than to confirm or eliminate a suspected condition.

A classic study of circumstances under which skull X-rays are ordered for head injuries is very revealing in this context. R. S. Bell and J. W. Loop[19] studied hundreds of patients who were brought to a hospital with apparent skull injuries and were subsequently X-rayed. They found that patients observed to have symptoms of confusion, drowsiness, headaches, visual disturbance, blood clots, lacerations, and swelling but no other symptoms, rarely had skull fractures. Out of 435 patients with some of the above symptoms who were X-rayed, only one (0.2%) had a fractured skull. However, among 1,065 patients having additional symptoms, such as unconsciousness for more than five minutes and discharge from the ears, etc., 93 (8.6%) had skull fractures.

Research on how to reduce the frequency of skull X-rays in emergency rooms has been conducted with financial help from the U.S. Department of Health and Human Services.[20] These studies are helpful to physicians and radiologists by providing information that can make their judgments less intuitive and more scientific in the future.

Once a legitimate decision is made by a physician or a dentist to order an X-ray examination, concern shifts to the skill with which appropriate equipment is used to perform a medically useful examination with a minimum amount of exposure. Two major factors contribute most to increasing the significant exposures of the reproductive organs to unnecessary X-rays. One factor is the failure to restrict the X-ray beam to the size of the X-ray film or to a smaller size. It is known that proper restriction of the X-ray beam size can result in significant reduction in the dose to the reproductive organs. Another factor that increases the dose received by the reproductive organs is the failure to use lead shielding to protect these organs from the main X-ray beam. It is estimated that with proper shielding, a 75 percent reduction in the significant dose to the male reproductive organs is possible.[21,22]

Equipment and techniques have improved tremendously over the years. The complexity of maintaining good facilities demands that they be staffed by those with adequate training and that they be properly supervised. Facilities supervised by physicians who specialize in the field of radiology have generally been operated with more skill and care than small facilities in the offices of nonradiologists.

CHAPTER

III

More about Diagnostic X-rays and Their Alternatives

Since the discovery of the X-ray in 1895, X-rays have been used repeatedly for the detection of broken bones, metallic objects, and gall or kidney stones, for example. In the years between 1895 and the present, X-ray diagnostics has developed into an increasingly fascinating and sophisticated science.

WHAT ARE X-RAYS?

To scientists, X-rays, like visible light and radio waves, are bundles of energy that move at the speed of light and carry electric and magnetic fields. Because X-rays are more energetic than light, they can penetrate material and collide with some of the atoms of which the material is composed. These collisions can result in the separation of an electron from an atom, or in ionization; thus X-rays, like gamma, beta, and alpha rays, are classified as ionizing radiation. When ionization occurs in the atoms of living tissue, it can produce biological damage.

If a section of a human body is placed in front of a beam of X-rays, some of the X-rays will pass through while others will be absorbed or scattered inside the body. Denser materials, such as bone, absorb X-rays more readily than surrounding tissues. When the X-ray beam exposes photographic film or a fluoroscopic screen, the shadows of the denser parts of the body appear on the developed film or screen.

TECHNIQUES IN X-RAY DIAGNOSTICS

The scope of X-ray diagnosis can be expanded greatly when substances known as contrast media are used. Air was the earliest and easiest contrast medium to be used. A deep breath held during a chest X-ray fills the lungs with air. X-rays pass through the air so readily that the tissues surrounding the lungs show up easily. Thus any areas where the lungs do not readily fill with air show up as cloudy spots on an X-ray film.

While X-rays pass easily through air, they are absorbed by dense substances such as barium or iodine, known as radiopaque materials. These can be used as contrast media if introduced into the body before an X-ray examination is conducted. Radiopaque materials can be swallowed, injected into the general bloodstream, or introduced locally using a relatively new technique known as catheterization. In this technique, a plastic tube or catheter is inserted into a vein or an artery and guided through the blood vessel to the location of interest under X-ray observation. A contrast medium can then be passed through the catheter. Taking X-ray pictures of veins and arteries is called angiography. The blood supply system of almost any part of the body can be studied with this technique. Barium and air are often used as the contrast media in gastrointestinal examinations. The patient may swallow a chilled, slightly sweetened barium drink, or may be given a barium or an air enema.

Early X-ray scientists developed methods of projecting X-rays which pass through patients onto fluorescent screens that give off visible light when excited by X-rays. This method, known as fluoroscopy, has enabled physicians and radiologists to observe the motion of organs or materials inside the body by viewing a patient continuously. A radiologist can watch a barium liquid pass through a patient's esophagus to his stomach.

Early fluoroscopes gave off a dim green light when

examinations were performed in a darkened room. Examiners were required to spend about ten minutes of precious time adapting their eyes to the dark before concentrating on a dimly lit screen. Mass-survey chest examinations are often conducted with a photofluoroscopic technique, in which a fluoroscopic image is photographed and the photographic image is stored on a small film. In this case, fluoroscopy is used to aid in reducing the size of the X-ray film rather than to observe a process in motion. Although fluoroscopic and photofluoroscopic techniques sometimes provide important information which cannot be provided any other way, they take longer to perform and they often expose patients to more radiation than conventional X-ray examinations recorded on film.

Modern fluoroscopes, however, usually require significantly less X-ray exposure than the older models, because of the recent development of electronic image intensification systems. These systems amplify the light from the fluoroscopic screen and then provide a brighter image on a TV monitor. Newer fluoroscopes are also equipped with foot pedals that turn the X-ray tube on and off, as well as with switches that allow an examiner to record interesting views on X-ray film for later examination. If properly used, modern equipment can provide better information, while reducing patient exposure by factors of 100 or more.

The typical exposure to X-rays has also been greatly reduced during conventional X-ray examinations by the development of new high-speed X-ray films and improved development techniques. Phosphorescent screens which surround the X-ray film are now used for many kinds of examinations. These screens allow an image to be formed on the film with a much lower X-ray dose. Improved techniques and equipment have increased the usefulness of diagnostic X-rays far beyond the early days when X-ray examiners were limited to the observation of "bullets, bones, and gallstones."

Computerized X-ray techniques such as those used in CAT-scanning (CAT stands for Computerized Axial Tomography) and digital radiography are yielding much more detailed information about structures inside the body.

In conventional X-rays, the image obtained on the film is a shadow of everything between the X-ray tube and the film. Many overlapping organs and tissues, sometimes difficult to separate, often show up on the developed X-ray film. Because air, soft tissue, and bone absorb X-rays differently, the projections of various body parts on X-ray film have different intensities. It is usually quite difficult, however, to see the small differences between normal tissue and diseased tissue even when overlapping organs present no problem. Even with new film, image techniques, and X-ray tubes, certain kinds of diagnostic information simply do not show up on conventional X-ray films. Modern technology has overcome this problem. The CAT-Scanner employs a combination of ingenious techniques to detect slight differences between a lesion or tumor and surrounding tissue, regardless of which organs lie above or below it.

The CAT-Scanner uses a series of narrow, pencil-like X-ray beams to scan the section of the body being studied. The X-rays pass through the body and are detected by an electronic device that automatically stays in line with each X-ray beam. Typically about 160 scans are made at one position, then the source and detectors are rotated about one degree and the 160 scans are repeated. When the detector and X-ray tube have rotated completely around the patient, the scan is complete. The thousands of bits of information from the sensors are stored in the memory of a computer. This information is then processed by the computer to reconstruct an image that can be displayed on a television screen or in printed form. A single scan takes anywhere from a couple of minutes to a few seconds depending on the type of scanner and the extensiveness of the examination. In general the newer models of scanners are faster.

The CAT-Scanner has been lauded by physicians as the greatest advance in its field since Roentgen discovered the X-ray. CAT-scanning was originally developed to help visualize brain abnormalities such as hydrocephalus (water on the brain), cysts, tumors, and blood clots. Accident victims suffering from brain hemorrhages often require immediate surgery. CAT scans allow physicians to identify this condition quickly. The scanner also helps physicians to distinguish between strokes caused by bleeding and those caused by blood clots. Although the external symptoms are the same in both cases, the treatments are different. Newer units have been developed to scan all parts of the body.

Although some radiologists claim that the pencil-like X-ray beam exposes patients to less radiation than a conventional X-ray examination, the dose from a complete brain examination is estimated to be equivalent to that associated with a series of skull X-rays (2 to 4 rads).

Although the radiation risks for CAT-scanning and conventional X-rays may be comparable, the scanning method avoids the risks associated with the injections of contrast dyes needed in some of the conventional procedures. For example, hospitals with CAT-Scanners have drastically reduced the number of conventional brain X-rays, called pneumoencephalograms. In this particularly unpleasant procedure, spinal fluid is removed from the brain and replaced with air or gas. The gas acts as a contrast medium, enabling radiologists to obtain X-ray images of the brain. The aftereffects of pneumoencephalography include headaches, nausea, and vomiting, and the radiation doses are high (25 to 50 rads).

Another type of brain X-ray is angiography, in which a contrast medium is injected into the circulatory system of the brain to make it visible to X-rays. The substances used are known to be irritating to the body and the probability of complications and even death is considered uncomfortably high (about 1 percent). Here, too, the patient receives a considerable amount of radiation. CAT-scanning can help to reduce the number of angiograms ordered, because it can be used as a preliminary screening tool to determine if the more extensive angiography is needed.

The benefits of CAT-Scanners for some kinds of brain studies are widely accepted, and experts are hoping that the newly developed body scanners will contribute to the early detection of cancers and other diseases in internal organs.

Other techniques that will further expand the capability of X-rays as a diagnostic tool are on the horizon. Many of the recent and proposed developments will probably decrease the exposure of patients to potentially harmful radiation in a given examination. For example, new rare-earth intensifying screens, which are over two times more sensitive to X-rays than conventional screens, are now available. Widespread use of these new screens should make it possible in the near future to cut patient exposure in half without changing the quality of the X-ray image. However, as the capabilities of X-ray diagnoses expand, so do the number of different examinations to which a typical individual is likely to be subjected. It is estimated that since 1964 the number of people receiving medical and dental X-rays each year has doubled, and that in

1982 seven out of every ten Americans received one or more X-ray examinations.[1,2]

HOW X-RAYS ARE PRODUCED

X-rays are usually generated in a glass tube from which all the air has been removed. They are generated when a current of electrons (negatively charged atomic particles), measured in milliamperes, is stopped suddenly by a metal target. The speed at which the electrons hit the target depends on the voltage placed across the tube. Thus, increasing the voltage across the tube increases the energy of the electron current and produces a more energetic and penetrating beam of X-rays. Some of the less energetic X-rays leaving the tube are filtered out and absorbed by the glass walls of the X-ray tube.

During the time an X-ray machine is on, the voltage that produces the X-rays may vary in a regular periodic manner between zero and a maximum value. The maximum voltage is often referred to as kilovolts peak (1 kilovolt = 1,000 volts), or kVp. Diagnostic X-rays are usually produced at voltages ranging from 20 kVp for low-energy X-rays to 150 kVp for high-energy X-rays. At a given kVp the X-ray beam produced has a distribution of X-ray energies between zero and a maximum value, which is the same as the peak voltage impressed across the tube. The distribution of the

X-ray energies in the beam determines the quality or penetrating power of the beam. The quantity of the beam, or the total number of X-ray particles in the main beam emerging each second, depends on both the peak X-ray tube voltage and the current, or number of electrons stopped by the metal target each second. The total number of X-rays striking a patient being examined is proportional to the electron milliamperage and the number of seconds (s) that the beam is on. Although the beam quantity also depends on the tube voltage, or kVp, the total X-ray quantity is often measured by machine operators in milliampere-seconds or mAs.

Some of the energy contained in the electron current within this X-ray tube is used to heat the target plate which stops the electrons. To prevent overheating and damaging the target plate, many X-ray tubes contain a larger circular plate, which rotates rapidly while the electron current is on, thus distributing the heat over a larger area of metal. The whirring sound of this rotating plate, or anode, is what one usually hears when an X-ray tube is on.

Since many of the lower-energy X-rays in a beam do not penetrate tissue very well, they do not pass through enough tissue to contribute to an X-ray picture. Many of these low-energy X-rays, however, are absorbed by the outer layers of skin and could cause needless damage. For all but a few types of diagnostic examinations the useless low-energy X-rays are usually filtered out of the beam by placing a sheet of aluminum which is 2 to 3 millimeters thick (about one-tenth of an inch) between the X-ray tube and the patient. This filter improves the "quality" of the X-ray beam produced by the tube.

An operator of a diagnostic X-ray machine can determine the beam quantity by adjusting dials to give a desired peak X-ray tube voltage (kVp), electron current milliamperage (mA), and time in seconds (s) for the voltage to be impressed on the tube. The beam quality varies with the voltage and current settings, as well as with the adjustment of the thickness of the metal filter. An operator will usually choose a different combination of kVp, mAs, and filtration, depending on the type of examination and the size of the patient.

NEW ALTERNATIVES TO X-RAYS: ULTRASOUND, THERMOGRAPHY, AND NUCLEAR SCANNING

Several relatively new technologies enable radiologists to obtain pictorial images of body structures. Methods known as ultrasonics, thermography, and nuclear scans are beginning to replace X-ray examinations in some cases.

In recent years the use of ultrasound (sound waves of frequencies above the range of human hearing) has become accepted as a major diagnostic tool. Since

1970 the sales of ultrasonic equipment have been increasing rapidly, and it is estimated that they will rival those of X-ray equipment in the 1980s.[3]

In ultrasonics, information about the internal structure of the body is obtained by recording the way sound waves are reflected from different parts of the body.

The same device that emits short pulses of high-frequency sound serves as a detector for the reflected pulses. If the sound source is moved continuously, an area of the body can be scanned. These reflected pulses can be transformed into an electrical signal that can activate a television screen and produce an image of the area being scanned.

Although ultrasonic scans can be used as a substitute for X-rays for certain kinds of examinations, they yield different information. The boundaries between different types of soft tissue can be highlighted with ultrasonics, and characteristics of blood flow can be studied. However, X-rays are still better for the visualization of anatomic structures such as bones.

So far, the most popular applications of medical ultrasonics lie in the diagnosis of heart abnormalities, eye conditions, arterial blood flow, and brain problems caused by tumors, cysts, or hemorrhages.

The use of ultrasonics in diagnosing problems in pregnancy is also becoming more common. Ultrasound has been used extensively on pregnant women as a replacement for pelvimetry and other fetal examinations. The amniotic fluid surrounding the fetus is an excellent transmitter of ultrasound, while the fetus serves as a reflector. This allows physicians to use ultrasound to view on a television screen an image of a developing child. Ultrasonic scanning of the uterus can be used to detect pregnancy as early as the sixth week, to determine the number and size of fetuses and the fetal position. Ultrasound has also been used to monitor the position of a needle in cases where it is desirable to withdraw some amniotic fluid for further study and to detect large fetal deformities. A major reason for the popularity of ultrasonic scans in pregnancy is the assumption that ultrasound, unlike X-rays, does not cause fetal damage.

Even though no studies have yet revealed any biological damage in humans from exposure to diagnostic ultrasound, it is a form of energy being transmitted through tissues, and like X-rays, it may eventually be proved harmful. When X-ray diagnosis was first used, practitioners were not aware of the subtle, long-term genetic and cancer-producing potential of low-intensity X-ray beams. Many of the effects of low-level radiation are not apparent until fifteen or more years after a person has been exposed to it. This may also prove true for ultrasound, but we are hoping that it will not and that ultrasonic diagnostics will at least provide a risk-free alternative to X-rays for certain procedures— especially those now exposing pregnant women to abdominal X-rays.

The full potential of ultrasonics has not yet been realized. Medical researchers are exploring a host of new applications for the technique, and engineers and physicists are designing and testing new equipment.

Another new development, thermography, measures the infrared radiation pattern resulting from temperature differences on skin surfaces. Commercially available thermographic systems consist of an infrared detector, camera, and display unit. The infrared detector scans the area of interest. Because the temperature patterns are already present and no energy is transmitted through the body, thermography is absolutely safe. Thermography is widely used in examinations of the breast and other organs, but, like ultrasound, it does not always yield the same information as X-rays. Thermography is used along with mammography to detect breast cancer. Unfortunately, thermographic scans are not yet as reliable as mammography for the detection of very small breast tumors. If they were, there would be no need to use potentially harmful X-rays.

Since the early 1950s nuclear scans have been commonly used for the detection of tumors. They are also used to study the amount of liquids located in organs, the rate of flow of liquids through organs or membranes, and the changes in internal organs during a period of time.

A nuclear-scanning procedure begins with the introduction of a radioactive substance into the body.

(A radioactive substance is one whose atoms give off radiation such as beta particles or gamma-rays, which are similar to X-rays.) The way in which a radioactive material passes through the body depends on the properties of the atom or molecule with which it is associated. Thus, after a radioactive material (or tracer) is introduced into the body, its location can be determined by a detector, which scans over the body and records how many beta or gamma particles are being emitted at each location. The number of particles at each scanning location can be transformed into a spot on a photographic film or a television camera, where the brightness of the dot will be proportional to the number of particles detected. If a tumor or an abnormal growth exists in an organ, more or fewer molecules of a particular radioactive chemical may tend to accumulate there than in the surrounding tissue, and the tumor would show up as a bright or dim spot on the scan picture. Since there are many different types of radioactive elements, almost any kind of molecule can be "tagged" with a radioactive atom. Thus physicians who specialize in the field of nuclear medicine have many different tracer substances that can be used for a variety of nuclear-scanning procedures.

Since some of the radiation given off by the tracer substance is absorbed by the body, the risks associated with nuclear scans are similar to those associated with diagnostic X-rays. In fact, some scans deliver a considerable radiation dose to the organ being investi-gated. Therefore, nuclear scans cannot be considered safe alternatives to X-rays. Nevertheless, when a nu-clear scan is needed, it can provide useful information, and nuclear scanning will undoubtedly remain an im-portant diagnostic tool.

CHAPTER

IV

How X-rays Affect People

When a person is exposed to X-rays, the damage done to tissues and organs can be related to his or her radiation dose. Observations of people who have been exposed to radiation indicate that such exposures increase one's chances of developing a number of conditions in later years, such as cancer or leukemia. Developing embryos and growing children are more susceptible to radiation-related health problems than adults are. Some people, regardless of age, seem to be more susceptible to radiation damage than others. Parts of the human body—for example, the thyroid and the bone marrow—where cells divide rapidly, are more susceptible to long-term radiation effects than other tissues, for example, muscle. Because exposure of the reproductive organs of young adults and children may cause genetic damage, which affects the health of future generations, it is also important to minimize the exposure of the reproductive organs to X-rays and similar radiation.

In spite of the fact that scientists know more about the biological effects of penetrating radiation than they do about any other environmental pollutant, direct observations of the effects of exposure to low doses of X-rays are not completely reliable. Moreover, the processes by which exposure to radiation may lead to poor health in subsequent years are not fully understood. More information is needed before it is possible to determine accurately the risks associated with specific diagnostic X-ray examinations.

The major assumption that lies behind the estimated risks is that the probability of long-term ill-effects due to X-ray exposure is proportional to the amount of radiation absorbed, no matter how small, and that even the seemingly low-radiation doses received from diagnostic X-ray examinations may increase the risk of developing these effects.

DETERMINING EFFECTS ON PEOPLE

The potential for danger from X-rays and other forms of radiation has often gone unnoticed in the past because the damaging radiation cannot be seen or felt.

Except for situations in which people are exposed to enormous amounts of radiation, signs of damage are not noticeable until some time after exposure, perhaps a number of years.

Three units are commonly used in discussions of the potential biological effects of X-rays and other types of radiation: the roentgen, the rad, and the rem. The roentgen is an approximate measure of the radiant energy to which a person or object is exposed; the rad and the rem provide a measure of the amount of energy actually absorbed by an exposed object.

Although on a technical level each unit is defined differently, for the purpose of the general discussion in this book, these units can be used interchangeably. One roentgen, rad, or rem represents a fairly large amount of radiation when compared to the average natural background dose received annually. For example, the average whole-body radiation dose received from natural sources (background radiation) in the United States is about 0.084 rem per year.[1] Often millirad (mrad), millirem (mrem), or milliroentgen (mr) is used instead. The prefix milli means 1/1,000, so that 1 rem = 1,000 mrems. Expressed in terms of the smaller units, the average whole-body dose in the United States due to background radiation is 84 millirems per year. (See Appendix A for a more detailed discussion of these units.)

It is estimated that the average resident of the

United States receives an abdominal dose of 78 mrems per year,[2] primarily from medical X-rays. Thus the average abdominal dose received from diagnostic X-rays is just slightly less than the abdominal dose received from natural background radiation in the United States.

EFFECTS OF MODERATE AND HIGH DOSES OF RADIATION

Experiments with animals and observations of people exposed to much larger doses of radiation than those associated with diagnostic X-rays have provided valuable information about effects of radiation on living organisms.[3] The known effects are of two kinds. One set of effects directly influences the health of the exposed individual. These effects are known as *somatic effects*. Another set of effects, which influence the health of the offspring of the exposed individual, are known as *genetic effects*, and are produced only when the reproductive organs (ovaries and testes) are exposed to radiation.

Somatic Effects

A study of American radiologists exposed to medical X-rays in their occupations and of two control groups consisting of other physicians indicated that, on the average, radiologists in the United States have a higher incidence of cancer than their medical co-workers.[4]

The tragic exposure of a large number of Japanese people to the very high levels of radiation from the atomic bomb blasts in Hiroshima and Nagasaki in 1945 has added greatly to our understanding of the harmful effects of radiation.[5] When very high doses of radiation are absorbed rapidly (when more than 50 rems are received at a rate faster than 1 rem per minute), such as those received by some Hiroshima victims, radiation sickness and in some cases death occurs within a few days or weeks after exposure. Other Hiroshima survivors, who received somewhat less radiation and lived for a period of years after the atomic explosion, had significantly more cataracts, cancers, and leukemia than an equivalent unexposed population. Pregnant women who received large doses of radiation and who survived the holocaust bore children who had an abnormal number of birth defects and a greater chance of developing cancer or leukemia. The number of miscarriages and stillbirths for this group of pregnant women was also significantly greater than average. Young children exposed to radiation suffered from many more health problems in subsequent years than adults receiving the same doses, although it was found that survivors of all ages who absorbed radiation had a greater risk of developing cancer or leukemia or of giving birth to deformed children in later years.

These studies of atomic bomb survivors indicate that when large amounts of radiation are absorbed rapidly by a person, the risk of subsequently developing cancer seems to be directly proportional to the radiation dose received. Thus a victim who absorbs twice as much radiation runs twice the risk of developing cancer in later years. This same proportional relation between high radiation doses and chances for developing leukemia and certain other long-term somatic effects has also been established for animals tested in laboratories, for children who were exposed to diagnostic radiation before they were born,[6] as well as for British patients who received large doses of X-rays while being treated for a spinal disease known as ankylosing spondylitis.[7]

Genetic Effects

There are no entirely convincing data available on the ways in which radiation actually damages the genes and reproductive organs of humans. For the most part, we know these organs must be damaged by observing the higher rates of genetic illnesses present in the children of people whose reproductive organs have been exposed to high levels of radiation. However, a great many experiments have been performed on laboratory animals (mice and fruit flies, for example) exposed to known amounts of radiation, and scientists believe the results of these experiments are indicative of the kinds of genetic damage incurred by humans. There is evidence that the reproductive material in human cells is somewhat more susceptible to damage than that in the cells of mice.[8] Thus it is believed that radiation of the reproductive organs of humans can result in offspring with a higher rate of mental retardation, cancer, ill health, and birth abnormalities. Except at very high doses, the amount of genetic damage done by radiation appears to be proportional to its dose and unrelated to the rate at which the reproductive organs are exposed. Harmful effects on the reproductive material (chromosomes) in human cells have also been observed directly when the cells are exposed to X-rays or other forms of ionizing radiation.[9]

It is felt that laboratory data obtained from irradiating mice provides the most significant information about the possible genetic effects of radiation on humans.

The Effects of Radiation on Living Cells

Cells are the building blocks of living organisms. Some scientists believe that both the genetic and the somatic damage associated with radiation exposure can be traced to the way in which radiation affects living cells. In any healthy organism some cells are dying while others are reproducing, replenishing, or increasing in number. Cells exposed to radiation often die or lose their ability to reproduce properly. Radiation loses its energy in passing through a cell by breaking apart some of the complex chemical bonds in the cell. As a consequence the chemical bonds characterizing the structure of the genes in the cell nucleus, which directs its reproduction, can be altered either directly or indirectly by the radiation.

The ability of cells to reproduce accurately is quite important, and it is very probable that the impairment of the reproductive ability of cells in the human body results in increased susceptibility to cancer and other diseases. The process of aging is also believed to be related to the reproductive ability of cells in an organism.

When a sperm or an egg cell from the human reproductive system is exposed to ionizing radiation, the arrangement of the basic genetic material, which contains instructions for the forming of offspring, may be altered or destroyed. These rearrangements, called mutations, may result in the failure of the cell to contribute to the reproductive process. A more serious consequence, however, is that such a damaged egg or sperm cell may produce offspring with physical, mental, or genetic damage. A number of illnesses and birth defects have now been attributed to genetic damage or mutations of one type or another.

It is well established that in humans the potential for harm from radiation exposure is greater for growing individuals whose cells most undergo rapid division to support growth. The embryonic stage is the most sensitive to radiation damage. However, in both adults and children some organs and tissues discard and replenish cells more rapidly than others. Organs and tissues that are more sensitive to radiation exposure than others include the thyroid and the red bone marrow, where blood cells are manufactured.

EFFECTS OF LOW DOSES OF RADIATION

The effects on humans of low doses of radiation (less than 25 rems) similar to those delivered during common diagnostic X-ray examinations are not immediately noticeable. Indeed, since the discovery of the X-ray in 1895, there has been an ever-increasing awareness of some of the more subtle long-term health effects of radiation. This fact is rather graphically illustrated by the way in which permissible doses for people working in the presence of radiation have declined over the years (see Figure 1). Since 1940 the permissible whole-body occupation dose has decreased fivefold. Currently it is believed that a person who is exposed to X-rays during a medical or a dental examination may have a slightly greater chance of developing cancer or leukemia in later years. Even if one of these illnesses develops, however, it would be impossible to trace its cause back to an X-ray examination, because

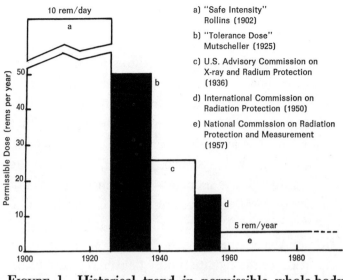

FIGURE 1—Historical trend in permissible whole-body occupational dose

people are also exposed to other cancer-causing agents, such as air pollution, food additives, and natural radiation. Exposure to such agents can also cause cancer, and it would be impossible to link an individual case of cancer to an X-ray experience.

As we have noted earlier, at moderately high doses (25 to 50 rems) and dose rates, a statistical relation between radiation exposure and various cancers and leukemias has been observed in both humans and laboratory animals. For low doses, however, it is more difficult to separate the effects of radiation on humans or laboratory animals from other influences in the human or laboratory environment. When conducting

43

experiments on the effects of very low doses of radiation on mammals, scientists need to study a very large group of animals in order to obtain valid results. This makes direct observations on humans quite difficult.

Until recently there was not much evidence that exposure to diagnostic X-rays affected human health. One recent study has shown, however, that exposure to diagnostic X-rays increases the chances of unborn children developing cancer or leukemia during childhood.[10] Although this study indicates that the probability of developing one of these conditions is in proportion to the radiation dose delivered to the fetus, the results are not conclusive, since it is easy to argue that the relatively poor health of those mothers who had X-ray examinations during pregnancy caused the increased susceptibility of their offspring to childhood cancers.

In 1972 a study *linking leukemia with the exposure of adults to diagnostic X-rays* was published.[11] In this study the development of excess cases of leukemia in adult males was traced to previous diagnostic X-ray examinations. For some unknown reason the females in the study group did not show a significant increase in leukemia.

Many more sophisticated studies will be necessary before the full story of how diagnostic X-rays are affecting humans is unraveled. At present we can make only judicious estimates, on the basis of other evidence, of how low-level X-ray doses affect humans.

How X-rays Affect People

In the laboratory there are quite strong indications that the response of mice to radiation dose is similar to the response of humans.[12] Both genetic and somatic radiation damage to laboratory mice and their reproductive cells have been observed at relatively low doses.

The Linear Hypothesis

Since it is difficult to establish an exact relation between biological damage and dose for low levels of radiation, many scientists believe that in the absence of concrete evidence it is most prudent to assume that ionizing radiation involves a health risk to the exposed person in proportion to the dose absorbed by that person. This is known as the linear and nonthreshold hypothesis. This hypothesis assumes there is no threshold below which radiation is harmless. Thus, *under the linear nonthreshold hypothesis any amount of radiation absorbed by an individual, no matter how small, involves some risk to the health of that individual and/or his or her potential offspring.* (See Figure 2.)

There is evidence, however, indicating that certain effects induced by high radiation doses are not caused by lower doses.[13] For example, many Hiroshima victims who absorbed large doses of radiation in their eyes developed cloudy films or cataracts over the eye lenses in later years. Cataracts were also induced in the eyes of laboratory animals exposed to large doses. On

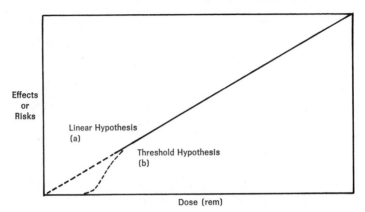

FIGURE 2—Relation between radiation dose and effect
using (a) linear hypothesis and (b) threshold
hypothesis

the other hand, animals exposed to lower doses of
radiation did not develop any cataracts. Cataract in-
duction appears to be a threshold effect in the sense
that there seems to be a dose below which radiation
does no detectable damage to the lens of the eye.
Many scientists believe, however, that genetic damage
can be caused at even the lowest levels of radiation,
that there is no threshold for this type of damage.[14]
Since the question of whether or not a threshold exists
for radiation damage is a matter of controversy, it is
interesting to speculate about the problem in terms of
the effects of radiation on the cells that make up the
human body.

When ionizing radiation, like an X-ray, passes
through a cell, the cell may be damaged. This damage

46

can either destroy the cell, impair its ability to reproduce, or cause it to reproduce with incorrect genetic information. The effect of high levels of radiation on an organism is serious, because many of its cells are damaged and destroyed. At lower doses fewer cells are damaged. In either case the number of damaged cells is roughly proportional to the amount of radiant energy (or dose) absorbed, no matter how small it is.

If individual cells have mechanisms for repairing radiation damage, then there may be a threshold dose below which radiation causes no permanent damage. However, the 1972 study linking leukemia in adult males to diagnostic X-ray doses suggests that if a threshold dose exists for adult males, it must be less than the doses delivered during some of the common diagnostic X-ray examinations. The relation between dose and effect at low X-ray doses has been a source of controversy for a number of years. Different dose-effect relations are discussed at length in a 1980 study by the National Academy of Sciences.[15]

The American College of Radiology has also taken the position that ". . . the prudent course at the present time is to assume that [radiation] effects may be initiated in a single cell and to assume that there is no lower limit to the radiation dose which might be considered injurious." In this book it is assumed that the linear hypothesis is a reasonable working hypothesis for protection purposes.

CHAPTER
V

Risks Associated with X-ray Diagnosis

The radiation risks associated with an annual exposure to diagnostic X-rays span a wide range, from examinations that may be comparable to regular cigarette smoking during a given year to those which involve negligible risks. Pregnant women, young children, and potential parents are usually subjected to more risks in a given examination than are other people. Additional risks are associated with certain diagnostic examinations involving the use of a contrast medium. These risks are caused by the introduction of the medium into the body and not by the X-rays.

In general, examinations of organs and tissues in

the abdominal regions involve significantly more somatic and genetic exposure than other examinations,
for several reasons. First, the abdominal region is filled
with relatively dense tissues, so more X-rays must be
used during these examinations. Second, a relatively
large film is used, thus exposing a large area of the
body to X-rays. Third, the reproductive organs are in
the abdominal region. Finally, special risks to the unborn child are involved when abdominal X-rays are
used on pregnant women.

HOW RISKS ARE EXPRESSED

In addition to radiation exposure, many other typical
human activities, such as taking drugs, riding in a car,
or smoking, entail risks. These kinds of risks are classified as somatic, meaning that they are potentially
harmful to individuals. Exposure of potential parents
to radiation and certain drugs involves genetic risks,
which affect only future generations. When both somatic and genetic risks are taken into account in considering diagnostic X-rays, estimation of the risks and
benefits becomes more complicated.

Until recently very little attention was given to obtaining numerical estimates of the risks or potential
for harm associated with familiar activities. Even in
cases where numbers have been assigned to risks, relatively few people use such information and change

their habits or conduct accordingly. A recent exception to this is in the case of cigarette smoking; the link between smoking and lung cancer deaths and other health conditions has motivated many people to quit smoking. If we are to begin taking more responsibility for our own health care, we must become concerned about the risks involved in various forms of medical diagnosis and treatment.

Several approaches describe the risks associated with various activities. Some analysts have attempted to devise a suffering scale for health problems that may result from certain activities. For example, using such a scale, a fatal radiation-induced leukemia would be much higher on the suffering scale than a skin cancer, which may be painful but which is rarely fatal. Another way to express risk is to place an economic value on induced disabilities or deaths. Such an economic analysis would add medical expenses to the loss of an average person's income from employment.

The easiest method to use in relating radiation dose to risk is to estimate the number of excess deaths that would be expected if a specified number of people were all exposed to the same hazard. This method has been used to link the probability of developing lung cancer to smoking cigarettes. For example, according to a study conducted by Drs. Hammond and Horn, about 130 people out of one million regular pack-a-day smokers will probably die of lung cancer each year.[1]

Risk estimates for various X-ray diagnoses, like the

risk estimate for smoking, must be approximate. Scientists do not know enough about the precise relation between absorbed dose and risks. Even if they did, the absorbed dose received from specific diagnoses depends on the techniques and equipment used to conduct each individual examination. Thus a reasonable way to express the risks involved in each type of X-ray examination is to calculate the risks with the use of good equipment and techniques and those using poor equipment and techniques. We can then assume that the average risk falls somewhere between these two extremes.

WHAT ARE THE RISKS OF DIAGNOSTIC X-RAYS TO YOUR HEALTH?

Estimating the risk of death from cancer or leukemia for various X-ray examinations is complicated by the fact that it depends on the age and susceptibility of the exposed individual. Also, each examination exposes different organs and tissues in the body to radiation. Areas of the body like the red bone marrow and the thyroid are much more sensitive to damage by radiation than muscle or skin. Recent scientific publications have described the relative likelihood that various critical organs will develop cancer after receiving a given radiation dose.[2] If we know the skin dose (amount of radiation absorbed by the skin), the voltage of the X-ray tube and type of filter used, as well as the organs in the main beam, we can use these figures to compute a cancer-producing or "effective dose" for a given X-ray examination.[3]

Effective doses for some common X-ray examinations conducted under average conditions are listed in Table 1 and Appendix C. A recent report published by the National Academy of Sciences, known as the BEIR Report, estimates using the linear hypothesis (see Chapter IV) that a whole-body dose of one rad or rem received by a million persons each year causes between 70 and 500 excess deaths from cancer annually.[4] If the effective dose concept is valid, then one rad of effective dose would affect the risk of cancer and leukemia in the same way as one rad of whole-body dose.

The average number of deaths per rad should be considered an upper limit, since it is still possible that discovery of a threshold dose in the future may indicate that some of the lower-dose diagnostic X-ray examinations involve little or no risk.

The effective doses and thus the cancer risks from different types of X-ray examinations vary widely. As shown in Appendix C, a lower gastrointestinal, or GI, examination conducted under average conditions may involve as much cancer risk as smoking somewhere between two and ten cigarettes every day for a year. On the other hand, average examinations of the extremities or dental examinations involve less risk than smoking even one cigarette a day. The cancer risk associated with the average U.S. background radiation dose of 84 millirems per year[5] is comparable to smoking about one cigarette a day. Typical examinations therefore span a wide range of maximum risk.

Thus GI examinations, which deliver the highest effective dose of any of the common procedures, may involve risks of fatal cancer comparable to the fatal lung cancer risks associated with regular smoking. (For details see Tables 1, 2, and 3.) On the other hand, a hip or thigh examination is about five to ten times less risky than a gastrointestinal examination, and the effective dose of about 100 millirems per year received from hip or thigh examinations is comparable to the average background radiation dose in the United States.

Risks to Future Generations

Although genetic risks to potential parents from X-rays are difficult to compare directly to the risks of smoking and other activities, information from the BEIR Report indicates that when the reproductive organs are included in the main beam, risks to future generations are similar to those encountered in submitting to X-ray examinations in the high-dose somatic category. Table 2 and Appendix C give data on the average male and female reproductive organ doses for various examinations.

TABLE 1: Average Effective Doses of Common X-ray Examinations (Somatic Doses)

A. *High-dose Examinations* (more than 125 mrads or mrems per average examination)

Mammography (breast examination)
Upper GI Series (barium swallow)
Thoracic spine (middle or dorsal spine)
Lower GI Series (barium enema, colon examination)
Lumbosacral spine (lower spine)
Lumbar spine (lower back)

B. *Medium-dose Examinations* (25–125 mrads or mrems per average examination)

Intravenous pyelogram, IVP (exam of kidney, ureter, and bladder)
Cervical spine (upper spine)
Cholecystography (gallbladder examination)
KUB (kidney, ureter, or bladder examination)
Skull
Lumbopelvic (examination of pelvis and lower spine)

C. *Low-dose Examinations* (less than 25 mrads or mrems per average examination)

Chest
Hip or upper femur (hip or upper thigh examination)
Shoulder
Dental (whole mouth or bitewing examination)
Extremities (feet, hands, forearm, etc.)

See Appendices A, B, and C for more details.

54

TABLE 2: **Average Dose to the Reproductive Organs from Common X-ray Examinations (Genetic Doses)**

A. *High-dose Examinations* (exposure of male gonads, more than 200 mrads per average exam)

Lower GI (barium enema, colon exam)
Intravenous pyelogram (IVP) (exam of kidney and ureter)
Lumbar spine (lower back)
Lumbopelvic (exam of pelvis and lower spine) *
Hip or upper femur (exam of hip or thigh) *

B. *Medium-dose Examinations* (exposure of male gonads between 10 and 200 mrads per average exam)

Upper GI (barium swallow)
Cholecystography (gallbladder exam) †
Thoracic spine (middle spine)
Upper GI (barium swallow) †
Abdomen
KUB (kidney, ureter, and bladder)

C. *Low-dose Examinations* (exposure of gonads less than 10 mrads or mrems per average exam)

Cervical spine (upper spine)
Skull
Shoulder
Chest
Dental (whole mouth or bitewing)
Extremities (hands, feet, forearms, etc.)

See Appendices A and C for more details.
* High category for females
† Medium category for females

55

TABLE 3: High Doses to the Uterus and Fetus

The following examinations of a pregnant woman may expose her unborn child to more than 4,000 mrads or mrems:

Abdominal aortography (examination of the main arteries in the abdominal region)

Lower GI Series (barium enema)

Celiac angiography (examination of the blood vessels in the abdominal cavity)

Upper GI Series (barium swallow)

Hysterosalpingography (examination of the uterus and oviducts)

Pelvimetry (examination to measure the size of the pelvis)

Placentography (examination of the placenta)

Renal arteriography (examination of the kidney)

Urethrocytography (examination of the kidneys, urinary tract, bladder, and urethra)

Cystogram (examination of the bladder)

See Appendices A and B for more details.

NONRADIATION RISKS

Some diagnostic X-ray procedures require the introduction of a contrast medium into the body in order to highlight certain organs or arteries. Contrast films are now quite common, and most contrast studies involve little risk. However, several types of studies involve added risks associated with the introduction of the contrast "dye" into the body.[6] The dangers of contrast-medium examinations include the potential for inducing a stroke or causing nerve damage when the dye is being introduced into the body. Some of the higher risk contrast X-ray examinations are listed in Table 4.

Because contrast examinations make up such a small percentage of the total number of X-ray examinations, the overall risks to the population from diagnostic X-rays are still due primarily to radiation effects.

A WORD OF CAUTION!

It is assumed that each and every X-ray examination adds directly to a person's risk in proportion to the effective dose to which he or she is subjected. Although

57

TABLE 4: High-Risk Contrast X-ray Examinations*

Type of Study	Method	Uses
Bronchogram	dye injected into lung bronchi (air passages)	outlines bronchial tree
Cerebral angiogram (arteriogram)	dye injected into carotid and/or vertebral arteries in neck	outlines blood vessels in neck and brain
Coronary angiogram (arteriogram)	dye injected into chambers of heart	outlines heart chambers, valves, and surrounding arteries and veins
Pneumoencephalogram (PEG)	air injected (as per myelogram); air rises into brain	outlines chambers and surface of brain
Pulmonary angiogram (arteriogram)	dye injected into pulmonary arteries as they leave heart	outlines blood vessels (arteries and veins) in lungs

* Source: *Talk Back to Your Doctor* by Arthur Levin, M.D., copyright © 1975 by Arthur Levin, reprinted by permission of Doubleday and Company, Inc.

it is desirable to keep the total radiation dose received by a person as low as possible, it is important to realize that the risks associated with each proposed X-ray examination must be considered in light of the potential benefits of that same examination. Thus, if a given X-ray examination seems necessary, a patient's past history of radiation exposure should not influence the decision to conduct that examination.

Don't forget to consider the substantial benefits of diagnostic X-rays. GI examinations as part of an annual routine executive physical may be completely unnecessary. On the other hand, in the presence of certain symptoms, the information obtained from a relatively "high" risk GI examination may save your life! In such cases the risk of *not* having a GI examination is greater than the risk of the examination itself.

Avoid routine examinations or prescribing X-ray examinations for yourself. However, do not avoid an X-ray examination if your physician can adequately explain why there is a real need for it!

In spite of some of the shortcomings of certain dentists, physicians, and radiologists discussed in this book, a qualified professional is probably a better judge of when X-rays are needed than you are. You have a right to expect any professional with whom you are dealing to provide complete answers to your questions about the need for a proposed X-ray examination. If, after reading Chapter VI, you feel that the practitioner's reasoning and diagnostic techniques are sound, you should abide by his or her judgment. If you are not confident about this judgment, by all means seek an independent one from another professional.

CHAPTER
VI

How to Minimize Your Exposure to X-rays

There are several ways to minimize your exposure to X-rays and still obtain legitimate benefits from X-ray diagnosis. First, you must discuss the risk-benefit question openly with your physician or dentist. A proposed X-ray examination might not be necessary. Diagnostic X-rays should be used only when the information gained will more than compensate for the potentially harmful effects of radiation.

It is not possible to say that you have or have not had too many X-ray examinations for your health. There is no firm evidence of a threshold effect for diagnostic X-rays; it is believed that the danger associated with each X-ray examination is in direct proportion to the dose received from it. Thus the overall risk to your health from diagnostic X-rays is considered to be roughly proportional to the sum of effective doses of radiation your body has received for all your X-ray examinations. The *additional* risk contributed by each subsequent examination is probably the same, regardless of the number of previous X-ray examinations you have had.

If there is a reasonable expectation that a proposed diagnostic X-ray will yield valuable diagnostic information which will influence the course of your treatment, it makes no sense to refuse it—even if you have had many X-rays. On the other hand, an X-ray examination that is not really necessary is not wise, even if you have never had a previous one. Sometimes a proposed examination is a repeat of a similar X-ray study conducted recently. You should refuse such examinations unless your earlier films are not available or unless the physician can convince you that there is a real need for a new study.

There are no known substances that can neutralize the effects of X-rays or other ionizing radiation after a person has been exposed. However, some research is being done on chemicals which may minimize the damage to cells if the chemicals are introduced into the body before it is exposed to radiation. It has been suggested that substances which act as antioxidants in cells may reduce the harmful effects of radiation. Thus, future research may show that if patients receive enough of an antioxidant such as vitamin E *before* a proposed high-dose X-ray study, the harmful effects of radiation might be minimized, although at present there is no firm evidence.

Your surest protection against unnecessary radiation exposure is to be able to assess whether the X-ray equipment and facilities are adequate. Finally, you must be in a position to evaluate some of the more obvious techniques and procedures employed by the people who operate the X-ray equipment. The amount of exposure can be decreased significantly if proper techniques and adequate equipment are used.

The information in this chapter is intended to help you evaluate your physician, dentist, radiologist, and X-ray technologist and their facilities.

THE DO'S AND DON'TS OF SUBMITTING TO X-RAYS

1. *Ask the physician, dentist, or radiologist who proposes an X-ray examination to explain what identifiable benefit will result from it.*

The following examinations are of special concern because they involve relatively high overall radiation doses:

1. Mammography (breast examination)
2. Gastrointestinal examinations (upper or lower)
3. Thoracic spine (middle or dorsal spine)
4. Lumbosacral spine (lower spine)
5. Lumbar spine (lower back)
6. Intravenous pyelogram (IVP) (kidney, ureter, and bladder)
7. Cervical spine (upper spine)
8. Cholecystography (gallbladder)
9. KUB (kidney, ureter, or bladder)
10. Skull
11. Pelvis
12. Hip or upper femur (hip or upper thigh)
13. Any fluoroscopic procedure (used to visualize motion)

On the average the following examinations involve a significantly smaller dose than those listed above:

1. Chest
2. Shoulder
3. Dental
4. Extremities (hand, foot, elbow, knee, etc.)

The need to question a practitioner about the benefit of a proposed examination in the low-dose group is less important than in the high-dose group. However, the professional organizations such as the American

How to Minimize Your Exposure to X-rays

College of Radiology, the American Medical Association, and the Environmental Protection Agency,[1] have recommended that no X-rays should be taken unless clear clinical reasons exist which indicate that they will contribute to a diagnosis.

In addition to radiation risks, there is potential for harm associated with certain diagnostic examinations in which contrast dyes are used. The following contrast examinations involve significantly more risk than others:

1. Bronchogram (outlines bronchial tree)
2. Cerebral angiogram (outlines blood vessels in the neck and brain)
3. Coronary angiogram or arteriogram (outlines heart and surrounding arteries and veins)
4. Pneumoencephalogram (outlines chambers and surface of the brain)
5. Pulmonary angiogram (outlines blood vessels in the lungs)

You should make an extra effort to determine the medical need for any of these examinations before submitting to them.

2. Ask the practitioner if it is possible to use the results of previous X-ray diagnoses instead of taking new exposures.

65

Sometimes a repeat examination is necessary to observe changes in a condition. However, physicians and dentists may not use current films because they do not trust previous studies, because they do not want to bother sending for them, or because they have not been told that the films exist. Keeping a complete record of your own X-ray history on a form similar to the one shown in Appendix E can help you to keep your practitioner informed about available records.

Some hospitals and medical groups have a practice of not accepting X-rays from other facilities. This practice should be questioned.

3. *You should express special concern to your practitioner about the need to X-ray children.*

For several reasons the potential for undesirable effects is greater in younger patients. Children depend on normal cell division to support their rapid growth, and radiation is known to impair cell reproduction. Children have a longer remaining life expectancy, so that effects such as leukemia and cancer have more time to manifest themselves in later years. Since children are small, it is often more difficult to keep their reproductive organs out of the primary X-ray beam. Finally, children are potential parents, and genetic damage is of special concern for this group.

4. *If you are a woman and there is any possibility of your being pregnant, inform your physician or dentist. Do not wait to be asked!*

X-rays which place a ripening egg or developing embryo or fetus in the main beam should not be taken unless absolutely necessary. X-ray examinations of a pregnant or potentially pregnant woman should be delayed if at all possible. An X-ray examination to diagnose early pregnancy should always be refused since other pregnancy tests are available. Some practitioners will not ask you about a possible pregnancy for fear of embarrassing you, so it may be up to you to offer the information.

5. *If you are pregnant, you should avoid all X-ray examinations of the lower back or abdominal region unless there are strong indications of a serious condition.*

A list of examinations which expose unborn children to the highest doses is included in Chapter V, Table 3. As mentioned in Chapter II, routine X-ray pelvimetry—X-rays in pregnant women to measure the size of the pelvis (particularly the birth canal) — has been found to offer "no benefit" and considerable risk. You should require written justification and explanation for using it if it is "mandatory" before you allow yourself to be subjected to this type of X-ray.

Some of the other examinations to be wary of if you are pregnant (because they may include the uterus and unborn child in the main beam) are:

1. Lower GI (barium enema)
2. Lumbar spine
3. Thoracic spine
4. Lumbopelvic
5. Cholecystography (gallbladder)
6. Intravenous pyelogram (IVP) (kidney and ureter)
7. Upper GI
8. Hip or upper thigh
9. Any other examination of the abdominal region

You should avoid all X-ray examinations conducted during pregnancy to visualize the developing baby or size of the pelvis, if your physician performs them on a *routine* basis.

6. If possible, have a physical examination and a dental checkup before a planned pregnancy.

Hormonal changes during pregnancy increase the chances of certain health problems occurring. For example, women are especially prone to developing gum and bone disease during pregnancy. Knowing whether or not you are in good physical condition ahead of time is worthwhile. Then if a physician or a dentist recommends a diagnostic X-ray on the basis of a physical examination, you can complete it before your pregnancy.

7. *If other means of obtaining X-rays are available, avoid mobile units.*

Several knowledgeable organizations have been urging discontinuance of mass chest X-ray screening in the general population in X-ray vans, yet a few local groups may be still promoting these programs. Modern diagnostic techniques, such as the tuberculin skin test, and the decline in the incidence of tuberculosis and other lung diseases have made unnecessary most mass chest X-ray screening. Besides, the mobile X-ray units used often produce miniature films, a process that usually involves significantly more exposure than conventional X-ray machines.[2] Don't decide on your own to have an X-ray examination. If a chest or any other X-ray examination seems necessary to you, consult with a physician first rather than prescribe it for yourself.

8. *If you are a woman under age 50 with no symptoms or family history of breast cancer, do not submit to mammographic screening on a routine basis.*

As of August 1976, the National Cancer Institute (NCI) no longer recommends the use of mammograms as a screening tool for symptom-free women under 50 with no family history of breast cancer. However, all women should practice breast self-examination monthly (see Appendix G). Any woman with any of the following symptoms should have a mammogram (X-ray examination of the breasts) immediately: pain, lumps, or discharge in the breast area. According to the American Cancer Society, women without symptoms between the ages of 35 and 39 should have an annual mammogram if they have previously had breast cancer. Women between the ages of 40 and 49 should have an annual X-ray examination if they or their mothers or sisters have had breast cancer. Women over 50 should consult with a physician about the desirability of annual mammograms.

9. *Avoid fluoroscopy if your physician acknowledges that ordinary X-ray films will provide adequate information.*

The use of the fluoroscope is similar to taking an on-the-spot movie, and it exposes you to the X-ray beam for a relatively long time. The X-ray is viewed directly on a screen, and may be recorded on film or videotape. Thus, a fluoroscope should be used only to visualize movements or change. Although newer fluoroscopes are equipped with image-intensifying devices to give better images with less exposure, the exposure can still be considerably higher than that acquired from standard X-ray film. Standard X-ray films usually provide clearer images anyway, and have the advantage of providing a permanent record. When a fluoroscopic examination is being conducted, however, a physician will often expose the necessary radiographic films at the same time.

10. *Question the need for routine preemployment X-ray examinations.*

Employees who handle food or work with people are often required to have chest X-rays to screen for tuberculosis. Ask if a tuberculin skin test or other tests can be substituted. If your skin test is positive, a chest X-ray examination may be necessary.

Employers having jobs involving heavy lifting are in the habit of requiring lower-back X-rays; in such X-rays the reproductive organs are often placed in the main X-ray beam. This procedure involves more radiation exposure than a chest X-ray. One of the major purposes of lower-back examinations is to protect the employer from a legal negligence suit if you develop lower-back troubles on the job because of congenital deformities. If you must submit to lower-back X-rays for the record, previous X-rays should be acceptable. If none are on file, go to a well-equipped facility supervised by a radiologist, rather than to a mobile unit or a physician's office. Men who are still of reproductive age should request a lead shield to protect their reproductive organs (testes).

11. *Refuse to submit to dental X-rays as part of every routine checkup unless you have special problems or unless your dentist can justify the need for these X-rays.*

Although full-mouth X-rays (sixteen to eighteen films) are sometimes recommended for new patients as baseline information, dental X-ray examinations should not be performed routinely as part of a dental checkup. They should be taken only after a clinical examination of the mouth and a dental history have been obtained. Examinations performed to explore special problems typically involve only one to four films.

12. *If you change dentists or are referred to a specialist, request that your new dentist obtain any available dental X-ray records.*

Previous records can help your new dentist understand your dental history and/or problems without exposing you to additional X-ray examinations.

CHECKING OUT THE EQUIPMENT AND FACILITIES

1. *In general you will receive significantly less radiation exposure at a facility under the supervision of a full-time radiologist.*

For example, the 1970 X-ray Exposure Study conducted by the Public Health Service indicates that examinations supervised by radiologists in private offices or in hospitals typically involved less X-ray exposure than those delivered by nonradiologists in their private offices.[3] Mobile units with fluorographic equipment usually give about five to ten times more exposure than the better types of facilities.

A specialist who uses his equipment and facilities full time is usually better able to afford up-to-date X-ray equipment and adequate facilities. There are exceptions to this rule, of course, so the best procedure is to check for some of the more obvious characteristics of a good facility outlined in the remainder of this chapter.

2. Ask if the X-ray facilities have been inspected by any licensing agencies or professional organizations.

Radiation control agencies in most states conduct periodic surveys of X-ray facilities. Results of inspection surveys are sometimes open to the public, and you can find out how skin exposure rates from given X-ray tubes compare with those used at comparable facilities. Contact your State Radiological Health Agency for more information.

In addition, professional organizations such as the American College of Radiology may review facilities and procedures as a way to help promote professional standards among their members. You can ask what organizations have reviewed the facilities and practices at your X-ray establishment.

3. *At a medical X-ray facility look for or ask about the presence of a beam-localizing light and an adjustable rectangular beam restrictor located in front of the X-ray tube.*

If the area of the X-ray beam is not restricted to the size of the film or smaller, you will be receiving needless exposure. For example, studies have indicated that proper restriction of the beam size can result in an average reduction by about 65 percent[4] of the significant dose to the reproductive organs.

The beam restrictor is called a collimator and works like the iris diaphragm in a camera, except that the shutters which open and close are made of lead, and that it produces a rectangular rather than a circular beam. (See Figure 1.) The beam-localizing light is an ordinary light located behind the shutters. When the light is turned on, it is projected through the shutters and outlines the size and location the X-ray beam will have. Thus, the operator can adjust the shutters and aim the X-ray tube properly before turning on the X-ray beam. *The shutters should be adjusted so that the light beam is no larger than the film.* In many cases, particularly in X-raying of children, it is desirable to

74

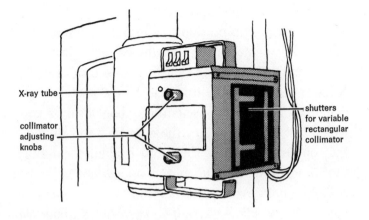

X-ray tube

collimator adjusting knobs

shutters for variable rectangular collimator

FIGURE 1—X-ray tube with shutters (collimators) for restricting the size of an X-ray beam

limit the X-ray beam to an area smaller than the film. If it is obvious that the light beam is much larger than the film or area being examined, *point this out to the technologist before the X-ray beam is turned on.*

In compliance with the Radiation for Health and Safety Act of 1968, HHS regulations require that machines presently being manufactured be designed so that the X-ray technologist cannot make an exposure unless the X-ray beam is collimated to, at most, the size of the film. Although in the latest machines the beam size is adjusted automatically, the light beam localizer is still used to outline the beam and to position the X-ray tube and patient properly. Very old X-ray machines do not have adjustable collimators or a localizing light, but are usually equipped with several nonadjustable cones that fit over the front of the X-ray tube. These machines can be used safely if the machine operator is conscientious about using a cone which restricts the area of the circular beam to about that of the film and if the beam is aligned carefully. *Operators have been known to work without adequate collimation to avoid poor exposures due to misalignment. Do not allow yourself to be X-rayed under this circumstance.*

4. *Avoid exposure to old-fashioned fluoroscopes.*

Before submitting to a fluoroscopic X-ray examination, ask about the presence of image-intensification equipment. Modern fluoroscopic equipment amplifies the X-ray image so that significantly lower exposures result. With older equipment the unamplified image is quite faint. The examiner must work in a darkened room and wear red goggles when the lights are on to adapt his or her eyes to the dark.

5. *If you are going to receive an initial mammographic examination, go to a facility which uses low-dose mammographic equipment.*

A breast examination should require no more than one rad of skin dose per film if proper equipment and techniques are used. Xeroradiography, which works on the same principle as Xerox copiers do, is rapidly replacing equipment requiring conventional X-ray film. (See the Glossary for a brief description of this process.) It is a good low-dose method. The equipment is easy to identify, because the technician is required to put an exposed cartridge into a large specially designed Xerox machine to obtain an image. No photographic films are developed.

If no xeroradiographic machine is available in your community, ask about the skin dose to the breast associated with the machine proposed for your examination. (High-dose machines are often used with no intensifying screen surrounding the film and with slower speed industrial X-ray film.) If the dose is more than one rad per exposure, try to find another facility with low-dose equipment.

6. *If you are to be X-rayed with a conventional dental X-ray unit, ask for one with a long open-ended, lead-lined cylinder on the end rather than one with a short, pointed, plastic cone.* (See Figure 2.)

The newer type of lead-lined cylinder, which is about eight inches long, is designed to produce a narrow beam and a minimum of scattered radiation.

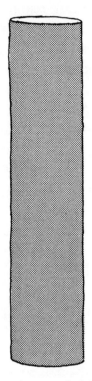

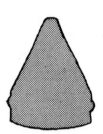

FIGURE 2—Short, pointed   Long, open-ended, lead-
    dental cone   lined dental cylinder

Scattered X-rays give you needless exposure without contributing to the quality of the image recorded on film. The exposure of the reproductive organs due to scattered radiation is about twice as much with the pointed plastic cone.

Your dentist can install long cylinders on his X-ray units without much additional expense. If he still uses pointed plastic cones, ask him to switch.

7. *There are several other important devices that help minimize unnecessary exposure and which are not likely to be visible to you. You may want to ask about some of these if the operator has time.*

A. *Fast film:* The use of ultraspeed X-ray film for medical and dental X-rays reduces your exposure by two-thirds or more compared to slower films. In some cases slower films which give greater resolution must still be used to obtain adequate information for a diagnosis.

B. *Electronic timer:* The newer electronic timers take the guesswork out of setting short exposure times, and thus minimize the number of retakes because of poor exposure.

C. *Metal filter:* The use of a metal filter, usually aluminum, is important in screening out low energy X-rays which are absorbed by a patient but do not contribute to the quality of the X-ray picture. In a few special cases the filter is not used.

D. *Metal grid:* If a moving grid is set directly in front of the film when medical X-rays are used, some of the scattered radiation which detracts from the image of interest is absorbed. This apparatus is called a Potter-Bucky diaphragm, or "bucky" for short. (A metal grid is not desirable in all types of examinations.)

E. *Image-intensifying screen:* For conventional X-rays other than those of the extremities (hands, feet, etc.) it is often advantageous to place intensifying screens directly around the film in the film holder while the film is being exposed to X-rays. The screens absorb X-ray energy which passes through the film and gives off additional light, which reexposes the film. Since the image on the film contributed by the intensifying screens is not as sharp as the image caused by the main X-ray beam, it is not always desirable to use screens.

CHECKING OUT THE X-RAY MACHINE OPERATOR

1. *In taking medical exposures, the operator should measure the thickness of the part of your body to be exposed and should consult a technique chart to set the tube current, voltage, and exposure time for each individual X-ray.*

Operators who guess or hurry through this procedure are more likely to take poor exposures. Repeated exposures due to sloppy techniques cause needless exposure to radiation. If the patient has an unusual muscle or bone density or moves during an exposure, the exposure will have to be repeated anyway. Careful operators have a repeat rate of less than 5 percent.

2. *A good operator aligns and restricts the beam carefully, especially when the gonads might be in the primary beam.*

For example, by taking an X-ray of the forearm of the patient in a sitting position and with the beam directed downward, the gonads can be included inadvertently in the direct beam. Proper alignment and use of a minimum beam size sometimes takes ingenuity. It is more difficult to keep the female ovaries out of the primary beam than the male testes. The operator cannot always avoid including a patient's reproductive organs in the direct X-ray beam. For example, hip, lumbar spine, and lower gastrointestinal tract examinations can all expose the gonads directly. *In many cases shielding the reproductive organs is possible, especially for men, and should be requested by all potential parents.* In some cases where the shielding obscures the organs of interest, shielding may not be possible. (See item 5.)

3. *A good operator uses extra care in alignment and a smaller exposed area of film with children.*

Children's organs are closer together and they are more sensitive to radiation damage. When exposing small children the operator should either use a smaller film size and narrow the beam, or just expose a small part of a larger film.

4. *Cooperate with the operator during X-ray exposures —do not breathe or move a muscle.*

This cooperation helps prevent blurred images and the need for retakes. Since it is difficult for infants and young children to hold still, to prevent a blurred exposure a parent or another adult may be asked to hold a child. *If you are asked to hold a youngster, request a lead apron. Refuse to help if you are pregnant.*

5. *If you are in the reproductive years or your child is to be X-rayed, ask for a lead shield for the reproductive organs unless the presence of a shield will interfere significantly with the information to be obtained by the X-ray.*[5]

Some examinations which directly expose the testes or male reproductive organs are listed below. Males of reproductive age or younger should ask for a gonadal shield for the following examinations:[6]

Lower GI (barium enema)
Upper GI (barium swallow)
Intravenous pyelogram (IVP) (kidney and ureter)
Lumbopelvic

Hip or femur
Lumbar spine
Abdomen
Sacrum and coccyx
Pelvis
Myelogram
Gallbladder

Even when the reproductive organs are not in the main beam, shielding can help reduce the amount of scattered radiation absorbed by the reproductive organs. Shielding of the male testes from direct radiation is possible in almost all cases, although it is often impossible to shield the female ovaries. (The examinations involving relatively high doses for the female ovaries are listed earlier in this chapter and in Table 3 of Chapter V.) Shields are often so easy to use that the extra measure of protection is very worthwhile. Some practitioners and operators, however, do not offer shielding to patients, to avoid frightening or embarrassing them. There are several types of shields including lead aprons, lead-lined panels, scrotal cups, flexible lead-lined drape cloths, and shadow shields (see Figures 3, 4, and 5).

Ask about shields before being X-rayed. Remember, however, that shielding of the reproductive organs should be used *in addition to* good collimation and *not as a substitute for* it. For example, in a lower-back examination of a male, an inch or two of extra colli-

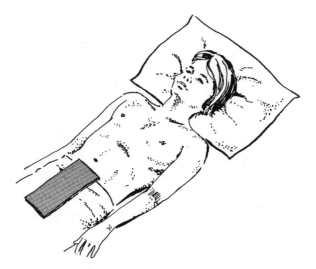

FIGURE 3—Lead panel-type contact shield

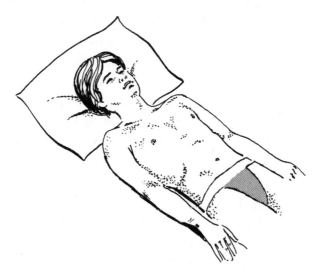

FIGURE 4—Scrotal cup in lead underpants

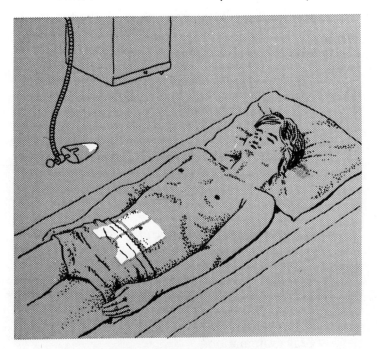

FIGURE 5—Shadow shield

mation at the lower end of the film can make a tre-
mendous difference in his testicular dose.

6. *Request that a lead apron be placed over your chest
and lap for dental X-rays and that a thyroid shield be
placed around your neck.*

In most dental examinations the reproductive organs do not lie in the path of the primary X-ray beam,
and a lead apron is not needed. However, a dentist

who aims the X-ray beam down through the top front teeth may be including the reproductive organs in the main beam. In that case, you should request a lead apron for yourself or for your children (who are also potential parents).

Since the thyroid gland is close to the X-ray beam, it may receive some scattered radiation. A flexible shield around the neck can reduce the radiation dose to the thyroid.

CHECK LIST OF QUESTIONS TO ASK

A. Questions everybody should ask medical and dental personnel:

- What benefit should I expect from the proposed X-ray examination?
- Are there clinical indications that an X-ray examination is needed, or is this a routine examination?
- Would you like to know about my previous X-ray examinations, and would it be possible to use the results of any of them?
- Is this X-ray facility inspected by any licensing agencies?

B. Questions everyone should ask medical personnel:

- Why is fluoroscopy necessary in my case?

- Is this facility supervised by a full-time radiologist?
- Are you able to adjust the size of the X-ray beam to that of the smallest appropriate film size?

C. Questions everyone should ask dental personnel:

- Do you use a long, open-ended lead cylinder?
- Can you provide me with a neck shield to protect my thyroid?

D. Questions for young adults and children who are potential parents to ask medical and dental personnel:

- Will my reproductive organs be in the main beam, and if so, can you provide me with a lead shield for them?

E. Questions for women who are or may be pregnant to ask medical and dental personnel:

- Do you know that I may be pregnant?
- Can this X-ray examination wait until later in my pregnancy or just after my next menstrual period?
- Will my uterus be in the main beam, and if so, can you provide me with lead shielding for it?

APPENDIX A

Units of Radiation Exposure and Dose

In order to understand how X-rays interact with people, it is necessary to have some understanding of the ways in which scientists measure the quantity of X-rays to which a person is exposed, as well as the amount of X-ray energy or dose that a person absorbs. Once the quantities associated with exposure and dose are defined, the potential effects of certain exposures or doses on human health may be discussed.

Defining appropriate units to describe the effects of radiation has proven difficult for scientists ever since the discovery of ionizing radiation. As a consequence, three related units of radiation, each slightly different from the others, have been defined. Respectively known as the roentgen, rad, and rem, they are often used interchangeably in describing X-rays that are striking an individual. This appendix is an attempt to describe important distinctions between these units of radiation.

EXPOSURE AND DOSE—WHAT ARE THEY?

The effects of diagnostic X-rays on the human body depend in a complex way on a number of factors such as the distribution of energies of X-ray photons in the beam, the total intensity or quantity of radiation, the distance between the X-ray tube and the person being X-rayed, the type and location of tissues and organs in the main beam, as well as the age and sex of the person being examined.

In an attempt to understand the relationship between the properties of a given amount of radiation and the biological effect on an individual, the concept of exposure was developed. Exposure is a measure of the number of electrons which are torn away from molecules when a beam of radiation passes through air. A positively charged air molecule and the negatively charged electron removed from it are referred to as an *ion pair*. The concept of radiation exposure is very convenient since it is easy to place an ionization chamber containing air in the path of radiation and record the number of ion pairs produced by the beam electronically. The common unit of exposure is the roentgen, named after Wilhelm Roentgen, who discovered X-rays in 1895. One roentgen is the amount of radiation necessary to produce 1,600 trillion ion (electron-molecule) pairs in one kilogram of air (1 kilogram = 2.2 pounds).

Although the exposure in roentgens is an easy quantity to measure, it is not always a good indicator of the effects of radiation on an individual. This is because tissue, bone, and other materials contain different types of molecules and have different densities from air. Furthermore, the processes by which ionizing radiation such as X-rays, or gamma rays, beta particles, or alpha particles lose their energy in passing through matter is different for each type of radiation. The energy absorption process also depends on the quality or energy distribution of the radiation as well as on the type of exposed tissue or bone.

The concept of *absorbed dose* was developed as a measure of the amount of energy dumped by incident radiation into a gram of material. The dose absorbed by a gram of skin or muscle can be much less than that of a gram of bone placed in the same X-ray beam. This is because the heavy atoms of calcium in bone absorb X-rays more easily than lighter elements abundant in tissue. Thus X-rays pass through tissue more easily and do not leave as much energy behind.

Absorbed dose, although harder to measure, is probably a better indicator of the biological impact of radiation than exposure. The most common unit of absorbed dose is the rad. Because the outer layers of material absorb X-rays readily, the exposure inside a person's body will be less than the exposure at the skin. The absorbed dose in the outer layers of skin is often referred to as the *skin dose*; X-ray energy deposited in a gram of bone, tissues, or an organ at a certain location inside the body is referred to as the *depth dose* at that location. High-energy X-ray photons have much more penetration power, and the depth dose corresponding to a relatively high-energy (100 kVp) diagnostic X-ray beam can be hundreds of times greater than that of a low-energy diagnostic X-ray beam (20 kVp).

Since the exposure in roentgens is the same as the absorbed dose in rads at the surface of soft tissue for medical X-rays, these units are sometimes used interchangeably. *However, in most situations a measurement of X-ray exposure in roentgens made with an ion chamber at the surface of the body is not the same as the dose or energy absorbed at various points inside the body in rads.* When other types of radiation such as alpha particles or neutrons are present, a unit called the rem is used. Rem stands for Roentgen Equivalent Man and describes the potential for biological damage resulting from a given dose in rads of radiation other than X-rays. *However, for X-rays, rad and rem always have the same value and can be used interchangeably.*

Units of Radiation Exposure and Dose

At present most researchers studying the biological effects of ionizing radiation on humans assume that its effects on a particular location in the body can be directly related to the absorbed dose in each gram of material at the location of interest. However, some effects may be related to the time period in which the dose is observed, or *dose rate*, as well as the total absorbed dose. Very high dose rates are known to do more somatic damage to individuals than the same total dose delivered more slowly. The relationship between genetic and somatic damage and dose rates for lower doses is not well established, and in setting radiation standards it is safer to assume that biological effects depend only on total absorbed dose (except at very high dose rates) .

The concepts of absorbed dose and dose rates are very powerful and useful. Our present state of knowledge is such that if a person absorbs a known dose at each location in the body within a specified amount of time, it is possible to set upper limits using the linear hypothesis on the effects the radiation will probably have on the person's health.

APPENDIX B

Exposures to Embryo and Fetus[1]

RANGE OF POSSIBLE EXPOSURES OF AN EMBRYO OR FETUS IN VARIOUS X-RAY DIAGNOSTIC PROCEDURES OF THE PREGNANT WOMAN

Diagnostic Radiography	*Dose Range in Millirads*
Abdomen screening	100–2,000 depending upon whether there are multiple films and/or fluoroscopy

---

[1] Robert Rugh and William Leach, "X-ray Effects on the Embryo and Fetus: A Review of Experimental Findings," Bureau of Radiological Health, FDA, United States Public Health Service, Rockville, Maryland 20852 (September 1973).

Exposures to Embryo and Fetus

Abdominal aortography*	6,000–20,000
Amniography	100 or more depending upon techniques used
Barium enema*	250–6,000 (higher with fluoroscopy and spot film)
Carcinoma of the cervix	To 6,000 if fluoroscopy is used
Cardiac series	5–50, higher with fluoroscopy
Celiac angiography*	2,000–20,000 (with fluoroscopy)
Cephalopelvimetry	See *Pelvimetry*
Chest	Single view, 1–10 or less; 5–70 or to 2,000 with fluoroscopy
Cholangiography	20–200 (films) or to 2,000 (fluoroscopy)
Cholecystography	20–200 (films) or to 2,000 (fluoroscopy)
Cystogram (excluding urethra)	500–1,000
Colon	See *GI series, lower tract*
Dacryocystography	1–10
Dental series	0 with lead and rubber apron
Esophagram (esophagogram)	To 500 with fluoroscopy
Extremities	Negligible (1 mrad)

* Denotes procedures which are high risk to the fetus because they may deliver 4 rads or more to it.

Femoral arteriography	1,000+
Fetal age	500–1,000
Fetometry	100–300
Gallbladder	See *Cholecystography*
GI series, lower tract*	350–6,000, higher exposure with fluoroscopy
GI series, upper tract	100–2,000, higher exposure with fluoroscopy
Hip (spine and buttocks)	300–700
Hysterosalpingography*	1,200–6,000; rarely involves pregnancy, upper exposure levels with radiopaque and fluoroscopy
Ileo-cecal study	100–2,000, higher exposure with fluoroscopy
Intestine, small study	100–1,000 with multiple films and fluoroscopy
KUB (kidney, ureter, and bladder)	200
Long bone series	50–200
Mastoid areas	25–100
Myelography	Minimum of 2,000 spot films and fluoroscopy
Nephrotomography	500–2,000
Obstetric examinations	500–2,000 if laterals and stereo included
Ocular foreign body detection	1–10
Pelvic, lower abdomen screen	80–500

Exposures to Embryo and Fetus

Pelvic pneumography	300
Pelvimetry*	600–4,000 (usually toward term)
Petrous pyramids	1–10
Placenta praevia	500–1,000 with contrast injection
Placentography*	300–7,500 with contrast injection
Pneumoencephalography	2–20
Polytomography (both ears)	3–30
Prenatal mortality detection	100–500
Pyelography, intravenous	400–2,000, multiple films and radio-opaque
Pyelography, retrograde	450–1,000, multiple films and radiopaque
Renal arteriography*	2,000–4,200
Retroperitoneal study	500
Salpingography	10–50
Sella turcica	1–5
Shoulder	Negligible
Sialography	1–10
Sinus series	1–10 (paranasal)
Skeletal maturity detection	Negligible (one hand, one knee, or more)
Skeletal series for metastases	50–200
Skull series	1–10 (average 4)
Small intestine survey	500–1,000 (without fluoroscopy)

Spine, lumbar (sacrum and coccyx)	214–2,000 with lateral and oblique views
Splenoportography	2,000
Temporo-mandibular joints	1–10
Urethrocytography (like KUB and cystogram but includes urethra)*	To 600 with films, to 6,000 with fluoroscopy, and to 20,000 with cine
Venocavography	1,000+
Ventriculography	2–20

APPENDIX C

Average Doses for Typical X-ray Examinations in Millirads

	Average skin dose per film (a)	Average integral bone marrow dose per exam (b)	Average no. of films per exam (a)	Estimated "effective" dose per exam (c)	Average gonadal dose per exam (d) M	F
Mammography	1500*	—	2/per breast†	250–300†	—	—
Upper GI	710	300	4.3	150–400	30	150
Thoracic Spine	980	200	3†	150–400	<10	<10
Lower GI	1320	600	2.9	90–250	200	800
Lumbosacral Spine	2180	200	3.4	70–250	1000	400
Lumbar Spine (LS)	1920	200	2.9	50–180	1000	400
Intravenous Pyelogram (IVP)	590	300	5.3	50–150	1300	800
Cervical Spine	240	50*	3.7	40–80	<10	<10
Cholecystography	620	100	3.3	25–60	5	150
Abdomen or KUB	670	100	1.6	10–60	500	500
Skull	330	50	4	20–50	<10	<10
Lumbo-pelvic	610	100	1.4	5–35	700	250
Chest (radiographic)	44	4	1.6	5–35	<10	<10
Dental (whole mouth)	910	20	16†	10–30†	<10	<10
Hip or Upper Femur (thigh)	560	100	3†	2–25†	1200	500

Shoulder	260	50*	2†	2–25	<10	<10
Dental (bitewing)	920	4	3†	<5†	<2	<2
Extremities	100	<10	2.7	<5†	<10	<10

References

(a) U.S., Department of Health, Education and Welfare (FDA) Publication 73-8047, *Population Exposure to X-rays U.S., 1970* (Rockville, Md.: Public Health Service, November 1973). Appendix III.

(b) International Commission on Radiological Protection Publication, No. 16, *Protection of the Patient in X-ray Diagnosis* (New York: Pergamon Press, 1970).

(c) Calculations reported by P. W. Laws and M. Rosenstein, "A Somatic Dose Index for Diagnostic Radiology," *Health Physics*, 35:629–642, November 1978.

(d) *Gonad Doses and Genetically Significant Dose from Diagnostic Radiology, U.S., 1964 and 1970*, U.S. Department of Health, Education and Welfare (FDA), Public Health Service, HEW Pub (FDA) 76-8034 (April 1976).

* *Ionizing Radiation: Levels and Effects, 1. A Report of the United Nations Scientific Committee on the Effects of Atomic Radiation*, pp. 162, 164 (New York: United Nations, 1972).
† Estimate by author from data reported by John K. Gohagan et al., *Early Detection of Breast Cancer* (New York: Praeger, 1982), Chapter 9.

APPENDIX D

Comparison of Radiation Risks to Lung Cancer Risks from Smoking

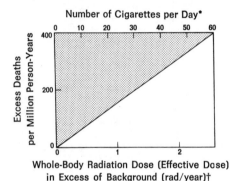

Number of Cigarettes per Day*

Comparison of excess deaths from lung cancer due to cigarette smoking and estimated average excess deaths from leukemia and cancer due to exposure to diagnostic X-rays and other ionizing radiation

---

* *The Consumers Union Report on Smoking and the Public Interest* (Mt. Vernon, N.Y.: Consumers Union, 1963), p. 34.
† *The Effects on Populations of Exposure to Low Levels of Ionizing Radiation.* Advisory Committee on the Biological Effects of Ionizing Radiation. National Research Council, National Academy of Science. National Academy Press, 1980. The cumulative lifetime excess of fatal cancers is estimated to be between 70 and 500 fatal cancers per million person-years per rad. The geometric mean of 107 deaths per million person-years per rad is shown on the graph.

APPENDIX E

Personal Radiation Record–
Diagnostic X-rays

Name .... Sex ....

Address .... Birthdate ....

Date	Physician or Dentist	Location of X-ray Facility	Type of Examination	Estimated Effective Doses*	Estimated Gonadal Doses*	Details (shielding, mAs, filtration, kVp, etc.)	Purpose of X-ray Examination

* See Appendix C for estimate of doses for various procedures conducted under average conditions.

APPENDIX F

Federal Agencies and Other Organizations Concerned with the Use of Diagnostic X-rays

A. **Federal Agencies Responsible for Radiation Protection**

Bureau of Radiological Health (Department of Health and Human Services)
5600 Fishers Lane
Rockville, MD 20857

As part of the Food and Drug Administration, BRH is responsible for protecting consumers against unnecessary radiation exposure, particularly from medical sources (including X-rays) and from consumer products such as microwave ovens.

National Institute of Occupational Safety and Health (Department of Health and Human Services)

5600 Fishers Lane
Rockville, MD 20857
This component of HHS is concerned with protecting workers from all on-the-job health hazards, including occupational exposure to radiation that might occur from the industrial uses of radioactive materials.

Environmental Protection Agency
401 M Street, SW
Washington, DC 20460
The function of EPA is to set standards which limit contaminants in the general environment, including radioactive pollutants from medical and industrial sources. This agency also regulates the use of medical and dental X-rays in federal health care establishments.

B. Other Organizations

American Academy of Dental Radiology
School of Dentistry
University of Florida
Gainesville, FL

American Association of Physicists in Medicine
335 East 45 Street
New York, NY 10017

American College of Radiology
20 N. Wacker Drive
Chicago, IL 60606

Federal Agencies and Other Organizations

American Dental Association
211 East Chicago Avenue
Chicago, IL 60611

American Medical Association
535 N. Dearborn Street
Chicago, IL 60610

American Society of Radiologic Technologists
645 N. Michigan Avenue
Room 620
Chicago, IL 60611

Health Physics Society
4720 Montgomery Lane
Bethesda, MD 20014

Health Research Group (Public Citizen)
2000 P Street, NW
Washington, DC 20036

APPENDIX G

Information about Breast Self-examination

Breast tissue is normally slightly lumpy. Women should examine their own breasts regularly in order to detect changes. If you feel a suspicious lump see a doctor as soon as possible. Many women put this off out of fear. Very few lumps are actually cancerous, but early treatment of cancerous lumps is important. It doesn't pay to wait.

Breast Self-examination[1]

Follow these rules:

1. Do this examination each month after your men-

strual period so that you can be familiar with your breasts in their normal state.

2. After menopause, check breasts each month on the first day of a new month.

3. See your doctor without delay if any unusual lumps or dimples are noted.

Examination Procedure:[1]

1. Lie down with the right hand under your head. Examine your right breast with your left hand.

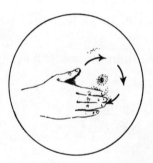

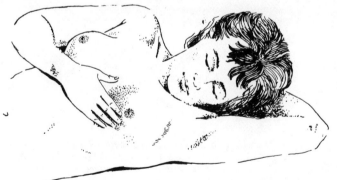

Push down gently with your fingers flat until you can feel the chest muscle underneath.

2. In your mind's eye, divide the breast into four areas, such as the four sections of a clock: 12:00; 3:00; 6:00 and 9:00. Starting at 12 (at the nipple), move your fingers clockwise from 12 to 3 and on around in a little circle. Then, move your hand up 2 inches and make another circle in the same way; then up another 2 inches, and so on, until the entire breast is covered. (If you notice a lump at, for example, 4 o'clock, you have a point of reference for yourself and your doctor.) Repeat this procedure with your left breast and right hand.

For films and literature on self-examination, write to:

The American Cancer Society
777 Third Avenue
New York, NY 10017
(212) 371-2900

---

[1] Reprinted from *How to Be Your Own Doctor (Sometimes)* by Keith W. Sehnert, M.D., and Howard Eisenberg, © 1975, by Keith W. Sehnert, M.D., and Howard Eisenberg. Reprinted by permission of Grosset and Dunlap, Inc.

APPENDIX H

*Diagrams of Organs
Exposed to the Primary
X-ray Beam in Common
Diagnostic Examinations*

The names by which doctors and X-ray technicians refer to various X-ray examinations are often confusing to the lay person. To help clarify matters for prospective patients, included in this section are illustrations depicting important organs and bony structures that are highlighted or which fall within the main beam in some of the most common examinations. The rectangles show the approximate size of the main X-ray beam for each exam. Beam size will probably vary somewhat with the technician taking the X-ray and with the size of the patient being examined. Some technicians also adjust the beam to a larger-than-necessary size, in order to avoid mistakes.

SKULL

highlights the brain

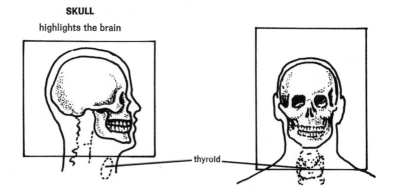

thyroid

Diagrams of Organs

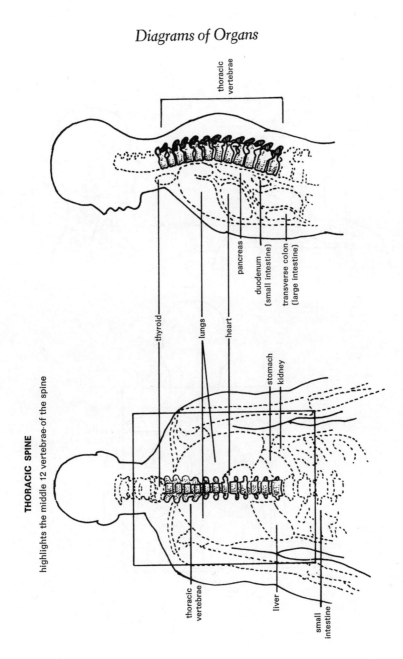

thoracic vertebrae

pancreas

duodenum (small intestine)

transverse colon (large intestine)

thyroid

lungs

heart

stomach

kidney

thoracic vertebrae

liver

small intestine

THORACIC SPINE

highlights the middle 12 vertebrae of the spine

CERVICAL SPINE

highlights the upper seven vertebrae of the spine

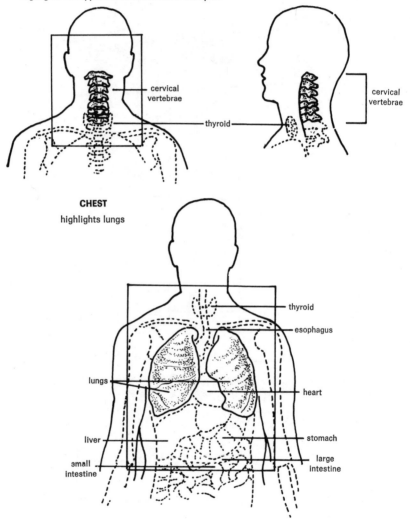

cervical vertebrae

thyroid

cervical vertebrae

CHEST

highlights lungs

thyroid

esophagus

lungs

heart

liver

stomach

small intestine

large intestine

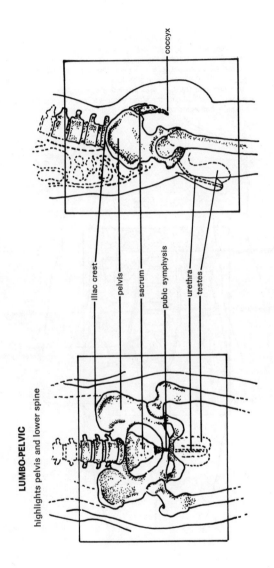

LUMBO-PELVIC
highlights pelvis and lower spine

coccyx

iliac crest
pelvis
sacrum
pubic symphysis
urethra
testes

Abdominal exams include the following:

Retrograde pyelogram — highlights kidney, urethra, or bladder

Lumbosacral spine — highlights the lower part of the spine, which is rigid and is connected to the pelvis, and the first few sacral vertebrae

KUB — highlights kidneys, ureter, and bladder

Intravenous pyelogram (IVP) — highlights kidneys

Renal arteriogram — highlights the blood vessels in and near the kidneys

Barium enema — highlights colon and lower gastrointestinal tract

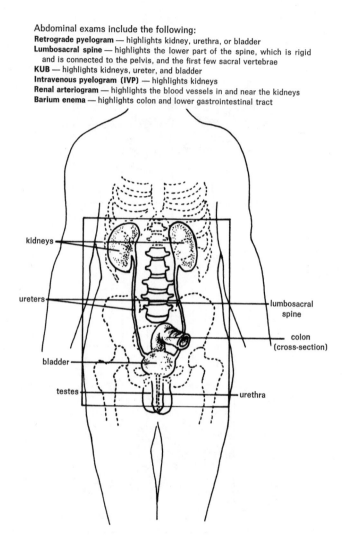

Diagrams of Organs

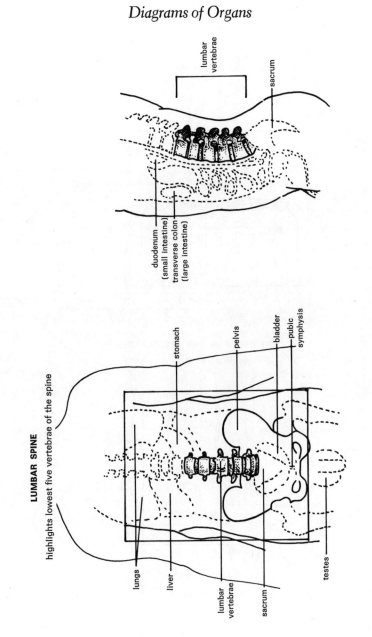

lumbar vertebrae

sacrum

duodenum (small intestine)
transverse colon (large intestine)

LUMBAR SPINE

highlights lowest five vertebrae of the spine

stomach

pelvis

bladder

pubic symphysis

lungs

liver

lumbar vertebrae

sacrum

testes

117

SHOULDER

highlights one shoulder (small rectangle)
or both shoulders (large rectangle)

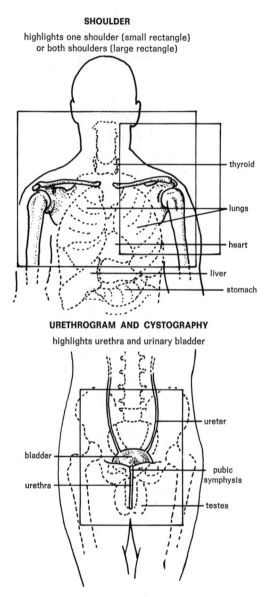

- thyroid
- lungs
- heart
- liver
- stomach

URETHROGRAM AND CYSTOGRAPHY

highlights urethra and urinary bladder

bladder

urethra

ureter

pubic symphysis

testes

Diagrams of Organs

RIBS

highlights ribs

esophagus
thyroid
ribs
liver
stomach
large intestine
small intestine

Note: *the heart and lungs lie behind the rib cage,
and are also exposed when the ribs are X-rayed.*

HIP

highlights one hip (small rectangle) or both
hips (large rectangle)

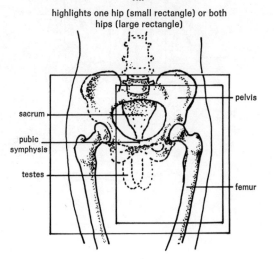

sacrum
pubic
symphysis
testes
pelvis
femur

119

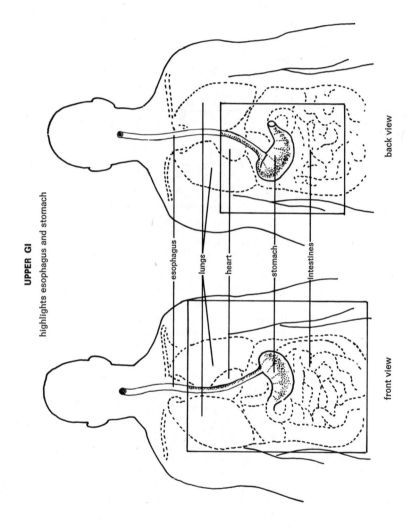

UPPER GI
highlights esophagus and stomach

esophagus

lungs

heart

stomach

intestines

back view

front view

Diagrams of Organs

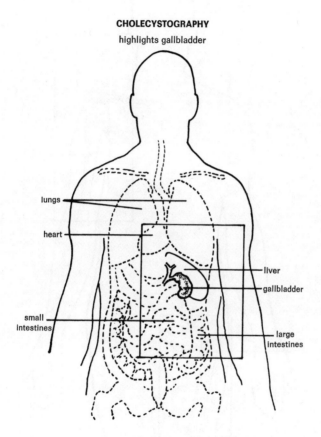

CHOLECYSTOGRAPHY
highlights gallbladder

lungs

heart

liver

gallbladder

small
intestines

large
intestines

back view

THE X-RAY INFORMATION BOOK

HUMERUS OR FEMUR

highlights upper arm or thigh

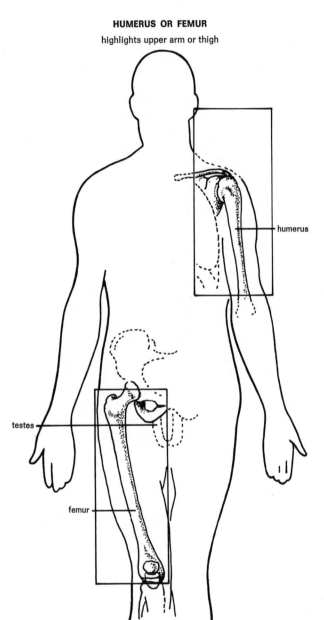

Diagrams of Organs

FULL SPINE

highlights entire spine; is used by chiropractors

- lungs
- liver
- pelvis
- sacrum
- heart
- stomach
- intestines
- testes

GLOSSARY

Terms and abbreviations used in X-ray diagnostics and radiation protection:

Absorbed dose—The energy imparted by X-rays or other ionizing radiation to a part of the body (usually tissue or bone) exposed to radiation. The special unit of absorbed dose is the rad, which represents 100 ergs of energy absorbed by one gram of material.

Absorption—The process whereby radiation is stopped and reduced in intensity as it passes through matter. Lead, which is denser than most materials, is a good absorber of X-rays.

Adaptation (Dark adaptation)—The adaptation of the eye to vision in the dark. The adaptation process is necessary for those operating old-fashioned fluoroscopy units, because the image on the fluoroscopic screen is quite dim.

Added filtration—Refers to the filtration (whether aluminum, copper, or lead) placed in the X-ray beam to absorb the less penetrating radiations which do not contribute to the quality of the

X-ray image. The use of appropriate filtration prevents unnecessary X-ray exposure.

Air contrast—The introduction of air into a selected part of the body because it does not absorb X-rays as do the surrounding tissues, and hence provides a contrast.

Air contrast study—An X-ray examination performed using air to outline soft-tissue structures within the body. The air may be swallowed, injected, or obtained from carbonated beverages, depending upon the circumstances.

Alpha particle—A form of ionizing radiation consisting of two neutrons and two protons. Alpha particles are often emitted from radioactive materials.

Angiocardiography—X-ray study of the heart and great vessels after the intravenous injection of an opaque fluid.

Angiography—X-ray examination of the blood vessels aided by the injection of a radiopaque contrast substance.

Anode—The positive electrode within an X-ray tube, toward which electrons are accelerated from the cathode. The kinetic energy possessed by the high-speed electrons is converted to heat and X-rays when the electrons strike the anode.

Anterior—Front.

Anterior posterior (A.P.)—An X-ray taken from the front to the back.

Aortography—X-ray examination of the aorta after injection of a contrast medium.

Apical (Lordotic)—A term describing a special projection used to obtain a better visualization of the tip of the lungs.

Arteriography—X-ray examination of the arteries aided by the injection of a radiopaque contrast substance.

Atom—A fundamental unit of which matter is composed. It consists of a heavy nucleus and surrounding electrons.

Autoradiography—A radiographic study whereby an X-ray film is exposed by radiations emanating from a radioactive material introduced into an organ of the body (or into a plant).

Background—A term used to describe the radiation present in the natural environment. It is produced by radioactive substances in the earth's crust, in water, in air, and by cosmic rays from outer space.

Barium enema (BE)—Barium is used as a contrast medium for an X-ray examination of the colon (intestines) or lower gastrointestinal tract.

Barium sulfate—Barium sulfate is a very dense material used in liquid suspension in the barium cocktail or drink used in some X-ray examinations involving the gastrointestinal tract. (*It must not be confused with barium sulfite*, which is very toxic.)

Benign—Not malignant. A benign tumor is one whose

growth does not spread beyond its original site and is rarely fatal to the host.

Beta particle—A form of ionizing radiation consisting of a fast electron. Beta particles are often emitted from radioactive materials.

Bitewing examination, dental—An X-ray examination of the molars by means of a small paper-covered film which has a small winglike paper flap that the patient holds in place by biting.

Bone marrow—A soft tissue constituting the central filling of many bones and serving as a producer of red blood cells. Bone marrow is especially sensitive to X-rays.

Bone survey—An X-ray examination of the bones. This survey is often used to determine the spread of cancer (metastasis).

Bronchography—X-ray examination of the bronchial tree, aided by filling the lungs with a radiopaque contrast medium.

Bucky—See *Potter-Bucky Diaphragm.*

Cancer—A growth (tumor) of abnormal cells which invades the body and may spread through the lymph or blood system (metastasize), thus causing severe illness or death.

Carcinogenic—Producing cancer.

Carcinoma—Malignant tumors derived from the skin, the membranes lining the body cavities, or certain glands.

Cardboard film holder—Used in certain types of

X-ray examinations. This type of film holder has no mechanism for intensification of the X-rays.

Cardiac catheterization—A procedure whereby a catheter or hollow tube is advanced along a blood vessel into a chamber of the heart for the purpose of obtaining pressure readings, for oxygenation determinations, or for the injection of contrast media.

Cassette—A kind of X-ray film holder containing intensifying screens mounted within front and back structures, which are hinged together. The X-ray film is placed between the intensifying screens in the dark room to prepare the cassette for use.

Cataract—An opaque body which forms in the eye, obscuring the transparency of the lens. Cataracts can be induced by high doses of radiation.

Cathode—The negative electrode in a tube where electrons are produced. It consists of one or two filaments and focusing cups.

Central beam (**Central rays**)—Refers to the X-rays in the center or the most intense part of the X-ray beam.

Cervical spine—X-ray examination of the seven vertebrae located at the top of the spine.

Cholangiography (**Post-operative cholangiography**) —X-ray examination of the bile ducts following surgery on the gallbladder.

Cholangiography (or **Cholecystography**)—X-ray examination of the gallbladder and/or bile ducts after the intravenous injection of a contrast material which subsequently appears in the bile.

Chromosome—Important rod-shaped molecules found in all body cells. Chromosomes contain the genes of heredity-determining units.

Chronic exposure—Irradiation that is spread out over a period of years. Those who are exposed to radiation on an occupational basis can suffer from chronic exposure.

Collimation—Restriction of the size of the X-ray beam.

Compression cone—This device is an attachment for use in fluoroscopy of the GI tract and serves to permit the examiner to apply pressure to various parts being examined, to displace some of the overlying structures, and to improve the examination.

Compression device—A mechanical means for reducing the thickness of a part of the body for the purpose of improving the X-ray examination. One type is used in IVP work (primarily for compression of the ureters) ; other types are used in fluoroscopy of the GI tract and mammography.

Cone—A round shield placed in front of the X-ray tube to limit the size of the beam.

Contrast—In radiology, contrast is defined as the difference (in density) between light and dark areas on the processed film. The contrast depends upon (1) applied kilovoltage, (2) filtration, (3) screen and film characteristics, and (4) processing solutions and techniques.

Contrast medium—A substance which, when introduced into a selected part of the body, absorbs X-rays differently than surrounding tissues to outline that part of the body more clearly. (See *Air contrast* and *Radiopaque medium.*)

Conventional therapy—X-ray therapy performed with equipment generating voltages up to 250 kilovolts peak (kVp).

Cosmic rays—Very energetic radiations from outer space, consisting of X-rays and charged particles.

Creep—The horizontal or vertical movement of fluoroscopic equipment during an X-ray examination.

Cystography—X-ray examination of the urinary bladder, aided by the introduction of a contrast medium.

Definition (detail)—In roentgenography, definition (or detail) refers to the sharpness of structure lines or contour lines on the processed film. Definition (detail) depends upon (1) size of the focal spot, (2) geometry, (3) filtration, (4) motion, (5) grain size of screens, (6) grain size of film, (7) emulsion thickness of film, (8) processing solutions, and (9) processing techniques.

Depth dose—The radiation dose delivered to a point at a given distance below the skin.

Dermatitis—An inflammation of the skin characterized by irritation, color change, lesions, and itching. This condition can be caused by overexposure to X-rays or other forms of ionizing radiation.

Discography—An X-ray examination of one or more intervertebral discs obtained by means of direct injection of a contrast medium.

Dose—A term used interchangeably with "dosage" to express the amount of energy absorbed in a unit of mass in an organ or individual. Dose rate is the dose delivered per unit of time. (See also *Rad*, *Rem*, and *Roentgen*.)

Dosimeter—An instrument which measures dose, for example, a pocket dosimeter.

Double-contrast study—X-ray examination in which both a contrast medium and air are used simultaneously (or in succession in certain instances) for the purpose of outlining soft-tissue structures within the body.

Electron—A negatively charged part of an atom or a molecule. When electrons strike materials at high energy, X-rays are produced.

Embryo—The term used to describe a developing human from conception until the fourth month after conception.

Encephalography—X-ray of the brain after the cavities have been filled with a contrast medium.

Expiration film—A term applied to an X-ray examination obtained while the patient holds his or her breath, after expiring (exhaling) the breath as much as he or she is able to do so.

Exposure—A measure of the number of ions produced in air by radiation. The special unit of exposure is the roentgen, which can be easily measured with an ionization chamber. Exposure should not be confused with dose, which is not so easy to measure and represents energy deposited in a certain amount of material.

Femur—Thighbone.

Fetus—The term used to describe a developing human embryo from the fourth month after conception to birth.

Film badge—A light-proof film packet used for estimating radiation exposure of personnel who work with X-rays or other forms of ionizing radiation.

Fluoroscope—A device in which a fluorescent screen is mounted in front of an X-ray tube so that internal organs may be examined when the X-ray shadow is cast on the screen. The fluorescent screen is coated with a special substance which emits light when exposed to X-rays. The fluoroscope is used when an examiner wishes to observe a continuous process, and the fluoroscopic image is usually amplified and displayed on a television screen.

Fluoroscopy—The practice of examining through the use of an X-ray fluoroscope. This technique is usually used to detect the motion of organs or materials inside the body.

Gallbladder (GB)—A membranous sac attached to the liver in which digestive fluid (bile) is stored.

Gamma rays—Photons or bundles of electromagnetic radiation of high energy which are usually more penetrating than X-rays. They are produced during decay of radioactive atoms.

Gastrointestinal (GI) series—An X-ray examination of the esophagus, stomach, and intestines. An upper GI series involves the ingestion of a barium drink for contrast. A lower GI series involves a barium enema for contrast.

GB series (Gallbladder series)—See *Cholangiography*.

Genes—Parts of chromosomes that determine the inherited traits of the offspring. Genes are contained in the nuclei of cells.

Genetic effects—Mutations or other changes produced by irradiation of the genes in a cell that might reproduce.

Gonads—Reproductive organs, or sex glands, consisting of male testicles or female ovaries.

Grid—A device similar to a grating whose purpose in radiology is to absorb scatter radiation which would impair the clarity of the image on the X-ray film.

    Stationary grid—A grid that does not move.

    Potter-Bucky Diaphragm—A grid that moves between the patient and the cassette during the exposure.

HVL (Half-value layer)—The half-value layer is the thickness of a specified material (usually aluminum, copper, or lead) required to decrease the dosage rate of a beam of X-rays to one-half its initial value.

Hard X-rays—X-rays of high penetrating power.

Hardness—A relative term to describe the penetrating quality of radiation. The higher the energy of the radiation, the more penetrating (harder) the radiation.

Head-clamp—A mechanical device attached to the X-ray unit in which the patient's head is held during an X-ray examination in order to reduce motion.

Health physicist—A professional who is especially trained in radiation physics and is concerned with problems of radiation damage and protection.

Heel effect—Refers to the unequal intensity of the X-ray beam, the intensity being greatest on the cathode side of the beam and least intense on the anode side of the beam. Some of this variation is reduced by use of lead apertures and shutters, which limit the periphery of the primary X-ray beam.

High-voltage X-rays—Voltage range from 140 to 250 kilovolts peak (kVp).

Hysterosalpingography—X-ray examination of the uterus and oviducts, aided by the introduction of a radiopaque contrast medium.

Glossary

Inherent filtration—The filtration effect of the materials (such as glass and oil) making up the wall of the X-ray tube.

Inspiration film—A term applied to an X-ray examination obtained while the patient inhales and holds his breath.

Integral dose—A calculated dose for a portion of the body, determined by (1) the size of the field, (2) the skin dose, and (3) the depth of tissue at which the dose falls to one-half the skin dose.

Intravenous—An injection into the veins.

Ion—An atom or molecule that has one or more of its surrounding electrons separated from it and therefore carries an electric charge.

Ion chamber—An X-ray measuring device in which gas is ionized in proportion to the quantity of X-ray energy passing through the chamber.

Ion pair—A positively charged atom or molecule (ion) and an electron formed by the action of radiation upon a neutral atom or molecule.

Ionization—The process whereby one or more electrons are removed from a neutral atom by the action of radiation.

Ionizing radiation—Radiation such as X-rays, and gamma rays, beta particles, and alpha particles which are capable of producing ions in matter.

IVP (Intravenous pyelogram)—An X-ray examination of the calices and pelves of the kidneys with opportunity for outlining the ureters and the bladder. Substances injected intravenously which are subsequently excreted by the kidneys make this study possible.

Kilovolt—Unit of 1,000 volts, used to describe the energy of X-rays. Most X-ray machines in medical use generate 20 to 150 kilovolt X-rays.

Kilovolts peak (kVp)—The maximum voltage impressed on the X-ray tube in kilovolts (1 kilovolt = 1,000 volts). The kVp determines the energies or "quality" of the X-rays in the beam.

Laminograms (Tomograms, Body-section films)—X-ray films of a selected plane, or level, in the body. Other tissues above or below the selected level are blurred-out by intentional motion of the X-ray equipment while the exposure is being made.

Lateral—X-ray examination taken from the side.

> **Right lateral decubitus**—Patient lies on right side.

> **Left lateral decubitus**—Patient lies on left side.

Lateral projection—The projection in which the X-ray passes through the part of interest in a transverse manner. Usually the side where abnormality is suspected is placed near the film.

> **Right lateral**—With the right side near the film.

> **Left lateral**—With the left side near the film.

Leukemia—A blood disease characterized by overproduction of white blood cells. The disease may result from overexposure of the bone marrow to radiation, or it may generate spontaneously.

Lienography—X-ray examination of the spleen after the injection of radiopaque contrast medium.

Linear hypothesis—The assumption that a dose-effect curve derived from data in the high dose rate ranges may be extrapolated through the low dose range to zero, *implying that theoretically any amount of radiation will cause some damage.*

Lordotic—See *Apical.*

Low-voltage X-rays—Voltage range up to 140 kVp.

Lower gastrointestinal (lower GI)—X-ray examination of the colon (intestine) aided by the use of a barium enema for contrast.

Lumbar spine—X-ray examination of the lowest five spinal vertebrae (bony segments).

Lumbosacral spine—Examination of the lowest part of the spine which is rigid and connected to the pelvis and the first few sacral vertebrae (bony segments).

MA (milliamperage)—The electron current flowing across the X-ray tube in milliamps (1,000 milliamps = 1 ampere). It determines the quantity of X-rays in the beam per second.

Malignant—Tending to become progressively worse and to result in death. As applied to a tumor, cancerous and capable of spreading locally or via the lymphatic or blood system.

Mammography—X-ray examination of the breasts.

mAs (milliampere seconds)—The product of the electron current in milliamps in the X-ray tube and the time in seconds that the current is on. The mAs determines the X-ray beam quantity.

Milliampere (mA)—The thousandth part of an ampere. The mA of the low-voltage filament current and the mA of the high-voltage circuit and X-ray tube are measured in radiology on milliammeters provided on the X-ray control panel.

Millirad (mrad)—One-thousandth of a rad.

Millirem (mrem)—One-thousandth of a rem.

Milliroentgen (mr)—One-thousandth of a roentgen.

Molecule—A group of atoms bonded together by electrostatic (chemical) forces.

Multimillion-volt X-rays—Voltages higher than about three million electron volts.

Mutation—A transformation of the gene which may be induced by radiation and may alter characteristics of the offspring.

Myelographic stop—A mechanical device used in conjunction with myelographic examinations in order that the fluoroscopy equipment will not touch or displace the needle in place for the lumbar puncture.

Myelography—X-ray examination of the spinal cord and adjacent structures after a radiopaque contrast medium is injected into the spinal canal.

Penumbra—In diagnostic radiology, penumbra refers

to haziness at the edge of an image due to the factors listed under *Definition*. In therapeutic radiology, penumbra refers to the irradiation of tissues beyond the projected bounds of the primary beam and is due in large part to scatter radiation.

Photofluoroscopic X-rays—Process by which X-rays are projected on a fluoroscopic screen so that the screen can then be photographed with conventional photographic film.

Photo timing—This is a method for timing X-ray examinations, the duration of the exposure being controlled by the amount of radiation which reaches a sensitive photo-tube behind the cassette. It provides a means for precisely reproducing densities on roentgenograms.

Photon—A bundle of electromagnetic energy. Each photon carries a fixed amount of energy. An X-ray beam consists of photons having energies in the X-ray region of the electromagnetic spectrum.

Pneumoencephalography—An X-ray examination in which spinal fluid is removed from the brain and replaced with air or another gas. This gas acts as a contrast medium.

Portal (port)—The port is ordinarily considered to be the region of skin through which the X-ray beam *enters* the body in therapeutic radiology. However, there is also an *exit* port, where the beam leaves the body.

Postero-anterior (PA)—The projection in which the X-rays enter the area of interest from the back (posterior) and exit through the front (anterior).

Potter-Bucky Diaphragm (Bucky) See also *Grid*— A bucky is a grid between the patient and the cassette which moves during the exposure and whose purpose is to absorb scatter radiation that would otherwise impair the clarity of the image on the X-ray film.

Projection—A term applied to the position of a part of the patient with relation to the X-ray film.

Pyelography—X-ray examination of the kidney after the injection of a radiopaque contrast medium.

Quality—A term used to describe the penetrating power of X-rays or gamma rays and is related to the energies of the photons in the beam.

Quantity—A term used to describe the number of photons in a beam of X-rays or gamma rays.

Rad—A special unit of absorbed dose equal to 100 ergs of energy deposited by ionizing radiation-like X-rays in one gram of matter.

Radiation—Energetic subatomic particles of electromagnetic waves which move at high speeds.

Radioactive material—A substance that contains atoms whose nuclei have excess energy which is given off in the form of ionizing radiation such as alpha particles, beta particles, gamma rays, or fast neutrons. A number of elements, for example, radium and uranium, are naturally radioactive. Others can be generated artificially in processes such as fission used in the generation of nuclear power.

Radiographic X-rays—Process by which X-rays are projected directly on film.

Radiography—*see Roentgenography*.

Radiology—The science of radiant energy and radiant substances; especially that branch of medical science dealing with the use of radiant energy in the diagnosis and treatment of disease.

Radiopaque medium—A material which absorbs X-rays and hence casts a shadow on the X-ray film or fluoroscopic screen.

Regenerative process—Replacement of damaged cells by new cells.

Rem—A unit of dose equivalent which is the same as a rad for X-rays.

Renal—At or near the kidneys.

Retrograde pyelogram—Examination of the kidney, urethra, or bladder after the injection of a radiopaque contrast medium.

Retroperitoneal pneumography—X-ray examination for the display of the transparent membrane lining the abdominal cavity. In this examination a gas is injected into the abdominal region for contrast.

Roentgen—The amount of radiation required to produce ions which carry a charge of .000258 coulomb in a kilogram of air.

Roentgenography—Photography by means of X-rays. (Roentgenography and radiography are commonly used interchangeably as essentially synonymous terms.)

Roentgenology—The branch of radiology dealing with the diagnostic and therapeutic use of roentgen rays. (X-rays are included, but radioactive substances are excluded in roentgenology.)

Rotating anode—Used in radiology for the purpose of dissipating the heat produced at the anode, thereby making possible longer exposures and greater tube life.

Sarcoma—Malignant tumors which arise in internal organs, lungs, bones, or connective tissue.

Scattered radiation—Radiation scattered in any direction by interaction with objects or within tissue.

-scopy—Suffix denoting the actual performance of an examination.

Seeds—Seeds are sealed sources of radioactive material used in radiation therapy for direct insertion into tumors. They are ordinarily left in place with no intention of removing them subsequently.

Shielding—Material interposed between a radiation source and an irradiated site for the purpose of minimizing the radiation hazard. Shielding is usually made of lead, which is dense and absorbs radiation easily. Shielding is often used to protect the reproductive organs, testes, or ovaries from the X-ray beam during an examination.

Shoulder support—A mechanical device attached to the X-ray unit when necessary in order to support the patient's shoulders and body when the X-ray table is placed in certain positions.

Sialography—X-ray examination of the salivary gland or duct after introduction of a radiopaque contrast medium.

Skin dose—A special instance of tissue dose, referring to the dose immediately on the surface of the skin.

Small bowel series—X-ray examination of the small intestine, using a contrast medium.

Soft-tissue film—A term for an X-ray examination performed with relatively low voltage for the purpose of providing optimal contrast for evaluating soft-tissue structures.

Soft X-rays—Soft X-rays are X-rays of low energy (kVp) and penetrating power.

Somatic—Pertaining to all body tissue other than reproductive cells.

Speed factor—With intensifying screens, the speed factor is defined as the ratio of the exposure required without screens to the exposure required with screens to get the same degree of blackening of X-ray films.

Spot-film—A spot-film is an X-ray exposure, using a

cassette, made during the course of a fluoroscopic examination.

Stereo—A term used for an X-ray examination in which two films are obtained in rapid succession but with a predetermined difference in projection in order that, usually with special equipment, the films permit visualization in three dimensions of an area in question.

Sterility—Inability (either temporary or permanent) to reproduce.

Superficial therapy—A term used in radiation therapy for treatment devised to maximize the effect of treatment on the skin while sparing the underlying tissues.

Target—That part of the metal anode or plate which faces the cathode and is struck by the beam of electrons. The X-rays are produced when the electrons strike the anode.

Target angle—The target angle is the angle away from perpendicular at which the electron stream from the cathode strikes the anode target.

Target-film distance—The distance from the X-ray tube target (anode) to the X-ray film.

Target-skin distance (TSD)—The distance from the X-ray tube target (anode) to the skin of the patient where the X-ray beam enters his body.

Teleroentgenography (Teleoroentgenography)— X-ray studies obtained with the tube at least six feet from the film, for the purpose of striving for parallel rays and minimizing distortion.

Thoracic—In the region of the chest.

Thoracic spine—X-ray examination of the middle twelve spinal vertebrae located above the five lumbar vertebrae and below the seven cervical vertebrae.

Threshold hypothesis—The assumption that no radiation injury occurs below a specific dose level. (See *Linear hypothesis.*)

Thyroid—The large gland located in the neck in front of the windpipe. This gland secretes a hormone which regulates body growth and metabolism.

Tissue dose—Used to distinguish between measurements made in air and in the body. Strictly speaking, tissue doses should be given in terms of absorbed dose (i.e., rads), but the roentgen unit is often incorrectly employed.

Tomography—Method for blurring out all parts of an X-rayed body except those lying in one plane.

Total filtration—The total filtration of the X-ray beam provided by both the inherent filtration and the added filtration.

Trendelenberg position—A position in which the patient lies with his head and upper body lower than his hips.

Tube—Usually refers to the glass tube within the head of the X-ray unit wherein X-rays are produced as

Glossary

the result of high-speed electrons striking a metallic target (anode).

Tunnel—A device, either part of a fluoroscopy assembly or part of a chest X-ray cassette holder, whereby a cassette can be protected from the X-ray beam before and after it is used to make a radiograph.

Upper Gastrointestinal (Upper GI)—X-ray examination of the esophagus or stomach, aided by the introduction of a radiopaque contrast medium.

Upright film—A term, sometimes applied to X-ray examination of the abdomen, in which the examination was obtained with the patient in an upright (or partially upright) position.

Venography—An X-ray examination of the veins, following injection of a contrast medium.

Ventriculography—X-ray examination of the ventricles of the brain after the injection of a contrast medium.

Volume dose—A calculated dose of radiation in gram-roentgens, based upon the air dose and the grams of tissue irradiated.

Xeroradiography (Xeros: dry)—A form of radiography performed without the use of X-ray film or fluorescent screens. A selenium-coated metal surface is substituted for X-ray film, and after exposure to X-rays, is dusted with calcium carbonate powder, thus producing an etchlike image. This is a photoelectric process and can be repeated as desired.

X-rays—Penetrating photons of electromagnetic radiation having wave lengths shorter than visible light. They are usually produced by bombarding a metallic target with fast electrons in a vacuum. These rays are sometimes called roentgen rays after their discoverer, Wilhelm C. Roentgen. In nuclear reactions, it is customary to refer to photons originating in the nucleus as gamma rays, and those originating within an atom but outside its nucleus as X-rays.

NOTES

FOREWORD

1. FDA Commissioner Dr. Jere Goyan, "X-rays: Get the Picture on Protection," *FDA Consumer*, December 1979/January 1980, p. 13.
2. Arthur C. Upton, M.D., "Low Dose Radiation Risks vs. Benefits," *Postgraduate Medicine*, 70:34–47 (1981).
3. *FDA Consumer*, December 1979/January 1980, p. 13.
4. Herbert L. Abrams, M.D., "The 'Overutilization' of X-rays," *New England Journal of Medicine*, 300:1213–16 (1979).
5. Report of State and Local Radiological Health Programs, Fiscal Year 1980 (Department of Health and Human Services, Bureau of Radiological Health, Food and Drug Administration).
6. J. R. Cameron et al., "Reduction of Patient Exposure," *Journal of American Dental Association*, 96:977 (1978).
7. *FDA Consumer*, December 1979/January 1980, p. 14.
8. R. O. Cummins and J. P. Logerfo, "Post-Traumatic Skull Radiography," *Lancet*, 471, August 26, 1979.

I. INTRODUCTION

1. A. W. Klement, Jr., C. R. Miller, R. P. Minx, and B. Shleien, *Estimates of Ionizing Radiation Doses in the United States, 1960–2000* (EPA, Washington, D.C., 1972), p. 98.
2. *FDA Consumer*, December 1979/January 1980, p. 13.

148

Notes

3. R. H. Morgan, Hearings before the Committee on Commerce, Science and Transportation, U.S. Senate. Oversight of Radiation Health and Safety, 95th Congress, June 1977.
4. *X-ray Examinations: A Guide to Good Practice* (HEW, Rockville, Md., 1971). BRH, p. 6.

II. MISUSES OF DIAGNOSTIC X-RAYS

1. Herbert L. Abrams, M.D., "The 'Overutilization' of X-rays," *New England Journal of Medicine*, 300:1213–16, November 21, 1979.
2. Report of the Secretary's Commission on Medical Malpractice (DHEW, Washington, D.C., 1973), DHEW Publication No. 73–88.
3. "Order More Diagnostic Tests," *Medical Economics*, September 30, 1974, p. 75.
4. W. O. Moms, *Dental Litigation* (Charlottesville, Va., Michie Co., 1972), Chapter 12.
5. Smith *v.* Yohe 194 A. 2D 167, p. 171. See also 162 *American Law Review*, 1295N, and cases therein collected.
6. E. F. Manny et al., *Pre-employment Low-Back X-rays: An Overview.* HHS (FDA) Publication 81–8173, August 1981.
7. Conference on Low-Back X-rays in Pre-employment Physical Examinations. Tucson, Az., January 1973. Summary Report and Proceedings (American College of Radiology).
8. *Population Dose from X-rays, U.S. 1964* (DHEW, Public Health Service, Washington, D.C., 1969), Publication No. 1519, p. 132.
9. J. L. McClenahan, "Wasted X-rays" (editorial), *Radiology*, 96:454, August 1970.
10. S. Bok, "The Ethics of Giving Placebos," *Scientific American*, 231 (5):17–23, November 1974.

Notes

11. "Consumer's Guide to Dental Health 1982: The Use of X-ray Examinations," *Journal of the American Dental Association*, 46C–48C.

12. "Dental Radiology: A Summary of Recommendations from the Technology Assessment Forum," *Journal of the American Dental Association*, 103:423–24, September 1981.

13. A. J. Nowak et al., "Summary of the Conference on Radiation Exposure in Pediatric Dentistry," *Journal of the American Dental Association*, 103:426–28, September 1981.

14. "Recommendations on Guidance for Diagnostic X-ray Studies in Federal Health Care Facilities," Environmental Protection Agency, 1976, EPA 520/4–76–002.

15. American Cancer Society Report on the Cancer-Related Health Checkup, February 8, 1980.

16. J. K. Gohagen et al., *Early Detection of Breast Cancer* (New York: Praeger, 1982), Chapter 9.

17. *The Selecting of Patients for X-ray Examinations*, HHS Publication 80–8104, p. 10.

18. Chest X-ray Referral Criteria, Panel Draft Report No. 1. Radiological Health Sciences Education Project, HHS Contract No. 223–78–6001, March 1980.

19. R. S. Bell and J. W. Loop, "The Utility and Futility of Radiographic Skull Examinations for Trauma," *New England Journal of Medicine* 284:236–39, February 4, 1971.

20. P. McClean et al., *Plain Skull Film Radiography in the Management of Head Trauma: An Overview*. HHS (FDA) Publication 81–8172, August 1981.

21. T. J. Withrow et al., *Possible Genetic Damage from Diagnostic X-irradiation*. HHS (FDA) Publication 80–8129, August 1980.

22. *Gonadal Shielding in Diagnostic Radiology*, DHEW (FDA) Publication 74–8028, June 1974, p. 3.

Notes

III. MORE ABOUT DIAGNOSTIC X-RAYS AND THEIR ALTERNATIVES

1. U.S. Department of Health, Education, and Welfare (FDA) Publication 73–8047, *Population Exposure to X-rays, U.S. 1970* (Rockville, Md.: Public Health Service, November 1973), p. 54.
2. Dr. Jere Goyan, "X-rays: Get the Picture on Protection," *FDA Consumer*, December 1979/January 1980, p. 13.
3. Jean L. Marx, "Diagnostic Medicine: The Coming Ultrasonic Boom," *Science* 186 (18 October 1974): 247–50.

IV. HOW X-RAYS AFFECT PEOPLE

1. U.S. Environmental Protection Agency (ORP/SID) Publication 72–1, *National Radiation Exposure in the United States*, prepared by D. T. Oakley (Washington, D.C.: Environmental Protection Agency, June 1972), p. 42.
2. National Academy of Sciences, National Research Council, *The Effects on Population of Exposure to Low Levels of Ionizing Radiation*. Advisory Committee on the Biological Effects of Ionizing Radiation. National Research Council, National Academy of Sciences. National Academy Press, 1980.
3. A. C. Upton, "The Biological Effects of Low-Level Ionizing Radiation," *Scientific American*, 246 (2): 42, February 1982.
4. R. Seltser and P. Sartwell, "The Influence of Occupational Exposure to Radiation on the Mortality of American Radiologists and Other Medical Specialists," *American Journal of Epidemiology* 81 (1965): 2–22; U.S. Bureau of Radiological Health, "Current Mortality Ex-

Notes

perience of Radiologists and Other Physician Specialists," prepared by G. M. Matanoski for the Division of Biological Effects Seminar, 12 December 1973.

5. *Sources and Effects of Ionizing Radiation: Report to the General Assembly*, the Scientific Committee on the Effects of Atomic Radiation, United Nations, 1977.

6. Ibid.

7. W. M. Court-Brown and R. Doll, "Mortality from Cancer and Other Causes after Radiotherapy for Ankylosing Spondylitis," *British Medical Journal* 5474 (1965): 1327–32.

8. *The Effects on Population.*

9. International Commission on Radiological Protection Publication 8, *The Evaluation of Risks from Radiation* (New York: ICRP, 1966), pp. 4ff.

10. A. M. Stewart and G. W. Kneale, "Radiation Dose Effects in Relation to Obstetric X-Rays and Childhood Cancers," *Lancet* 1 (1970): 1185–88.

11. R. Gibson et al., "Irradiation in the Epidemiology of Leukemia from Low Level Radiation: Identification of Susceptible Children," *New England Journal of Medicine* 287 (1972): 107–10.

12. U.S. Public Health Service (FDA), "X-ray Effects on the Embryo and Fetus: A Review of Experimental Findings," prepared by Robert Rugh and William Leach for the Bureau of Radiological Health (Rockville, Md.: Bureau of Radiological Health, September 1973), p. 2.

13. International Commission on Radiological Protection Publication 14, *Radiosensitivity and Spatial Distribution of Dose* (New York: ICRP, 1966), pp. 37ff.

14. Ibid., pp. 19–20.

15. *The Effects on Population.*

V. RISKS ASSOCIATED WITH
X-RAY DIAGNOSIS

1. *The Consumers Union Report on Smoking and the Public Interest* (Mt. Vernon, N.Y.: Consumers Union, 1963), p. 34.
2. International Commission on Radiological Protection Publication 14, *Radiosensitivity and Spatial Distribution of Dose* (New York: ICRP, 1966), appendix 4, pp. 74ff.; National Academy of Sciences, National Research Council, *The Effects on Population of Exposure to Low Levels of Ionizing Radiation*, Advisory Committee on the Biological Effects of Ionizing Radiation, National Academy Press, 1980; *Sources and Effects of Ionizing Radiation: Report to the General Assembly*, the Scientific Committee on the Effects of Atomic Radiation, United Nations, 1977.
3. W. Jacobi, "The Concept of Effective Dose Proposed for the Combination of Organ Doses," *Radiation and Environmental Biophysics* 12 (1975): 101–09; P. W. Laws and M. Rosenstein, "A Somatic Dose Index for Diagnostic Radiology," *Health Physics* 35 (November 1978), pp. 629–42.
4. *The Effects on Population.*
5. U.S. Environmental Protection Agency (ORP/SID) Publication 72–1, *National Radiation Exposure in the United States*, prepared by D. T. Oakley (Washington, D.C.: Environmental Protection Agency, June 1972), p. 42.
6. Arthur Levin, *Talk Back to Your Doctor* (New York: Doubleday, 1975).

Notes

VI. HOW TO MINIMIZE YOUR EXPOSURE TO X-RAYS

1. *Recommendation on Guidance for Technic to Reduce Unnecessary Exposure from X-ray Studies in Federal Health Care Facilities,* Environmental Protection Agency, EPA 52014–76–012. June 1976.
2. U.S. Department of Health, Education, and Welfare, Public Health Service Publication 1519, *Population Exposure to X-rays, U.S. 1964* (Rockville, Md.: Public Health Service, 1968), p. 148.
3. U.S. Department of Health, Education, and Welfare (FDA) Publication 73–8047, *Population Exposure to X-rays, U.S. 1970* (Rockville, Md.: Public Health Service, November 1973), p. 98.
4. National Academy of Sciences, National Research Council, *The Effects on Population of Exposure to Low Levels of Ionizing Radiation,* November 1972, p. 13.
5. Over the past several years, a number of organizations have recommended the use of shielding for the reproductive organs. These organizations include the American College of Radiology (ACR), the National Council on Radiation Protection (NCRP), the International Commission on Radiological Protection (ICRP), the National Academy of Sciences (NAS), the Bureau of Radiological Health (BRH), and the Environmental Protection Agency (EPA).
6. U.S. Department of Health, Education, and Welfare (FDA) Publication 74–8028, *Gonadal Shielding in Diagnostic Radiology* (Rockville, Md.: Bureau of Radiological Health, June 1974), p. 5.